MASTERING

BACH

FLOWER

THERAPIES

A Guide to
Diagnosis & Treatment

MECHTHILD SCHEFFER
Translated by Walter C. Schell

Healing Arts Press
Rochester, Vermont

Healing Arts Press
One Park Street
Rochester, Vermont 05767
Web Site: http://www.gotoit.com
Copyright © 1996 by Mechthild Scheffer

All rights reserved. No part of this book may be reproduced or utilized in any form or by
any means, electronic or mechanical, including photocopying, recording, or by any
information storage and retrieval system, without permission in writing from the publisher.

Note to the reader: This book is intended as an informational guide. The remedies,
approaches, and techniques described herein are meant to supplement, and not to be a
substitute for, professional medical care or treatment. They should not be used to treat a
serious ailment without prior consultation with a qualified health care professional.

LIBRARY OF CONGRESS CATALOGING-IN-PUBLICATION DATA

Scheffer, Mechthild.
[Erfahrungen mit der Bach Blütentherapie. English]
Mastering Bach flower therapies : a guide to diagnosis and treatment /
Mechthild Scheffer.
p. cm.
Includes index.
ISBN 0-89281-630-9
1. Flowers—Therapeutic use. 2. Flowers—Therapeutic use—Case studies.
3. Homeopathy—Materia medica and therapeutics. 4. Bach, Edward, 1886-1936.
I. Title.
RX615.F55S3513 1996
615'.321—dc20   96-5716
CIP

Printed and bound in the United States

10   9   8   7   6   5   4   3   2   1

Type design and layout by Virginia L. Scott

This book was typeset in Bulmer with Koch Antigua and Margaret as
the display typefaces

Healing Arts Press is a division of Inner Traditions International

Distributed to the book trade in Canada by Publishers Group West (PGW),
Toronto, Ontario
Distributed to the health food trade in Canada by Alive Books, Toronto and Vancouver
Distributed to the book trade in the United Kingdom by Deep Books, London
Distributed to the book trade in Australia by Millennium Books, Newtown, N. S. W.
Distributed to the book trade in New Zealand by Tandem Press, Auckland
Distributed to the book trade in South Africa by Alternative Books, Randburg

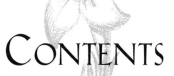

CONTENTS

A flower that opens makes no noise. On light soles beauty, luck, and heroism wander. Anything that is to have permanence in this noisy world of fake heroism, false luck, and untrue beauty shall come imperceptibly.

Wilhem Raabe

Whether the masses of millions—having material strength and means that appear so fruitful and unshakeable—will triumph in history will be due not to money, the sword, or power, but to the beginnings of hardly perceptible thoughts of seemingly unimportant people.

Dostoyevsky

PREFACE

This book is a continuation and addition to *Bach Flower Therapy* and should be read in connection with it. It contains a small but representative group of firsthand experiences with Bach Flower Therapies in Germany, Austria, and Switzerland. To all the friends of the Bach Flowers this book's practical applications will bring about encouraging insight and valuable recognition and it will reveal the wide spectrum of "flowers that heal through the soul."

The contributions* come from doctors and naturopaths who have introduced Bach Flower Therapy into their practices, as well as from a large circle of medically interested lay people who have used the Bach Flowers for self-discovery in their family circle or

. . . .
* Original letters and case studies are in possession of the Dr. Edward Bach Centre, German Office.

on their pets and plants. Many of them are participants in the Bach Flower seminars.*

In reading the hundreds of contributions I was deeply touched, and I would like to thank all those who have supported Edward Bach's idea of "healing through the soul" and with it the concept of human dignity in relation to illness and health.

After the release of *Bach Flower Therapy,* readers of that book recognized themselves in many flower descriptions, but found they experienced difficulty in deciding which flower to assign priority to in a given situation.

The practical diagnostic questionnaire supplied in the appendix of this book—primarily developed for Bach Flower Therapy—should, particularly for the beginner, facilitate the choice of a relevant flower combination. A shorter version can be obtained by doctors and naturopaths for their patients through the Dr. Edward Bach Centre.

For information and advice concerning the use and purchase of essences of flowers or regarding Bach Flower seminars, and for all other inquiries about Bach Flower Therapies please contact the following:

England

Bach Flower Remedies Ltd.
Dr. Edward Bach Center
Mount Vernon
Sotwell, Wallingford
Oxfordshire OX10 0PZ
England
Tel: 0491 39489/34678

. . . .
* The original Bach Flower seminars, the official Bach Flower Therapy continuing education programs, are given by the Dr. Edward Bach Centre, German Office, in Germany, Austria, and Switzerland.

North America

Ellon (Bach USA), Inc.
P.O. Box 320
Woodmere, NY 11598
USA
Tel: (516) 593-2206

Australia

The Pharmaceutical Plant Company
P.O. Box 68
Bayswater, Victoria 3153
Australia
03-7628577/8522

Martin & Pleasance Wholesale Pty Ltd.
P.O. Box 4
Collingwood, Victoria 3066
Australia
Tel.: 419-9733

An important note for the reader: The system of the thirty-eight Bach Flowers can act as an aid to self-healing, allowing you to take hold of transitory negative moods such as uncertainty, jealousy, faintheartedness, and others brought on by weakness of character. The goal of therapy is purification of the soul, self-realization, harmonious development, and greater personal stability. An indirect result is a lighter resistance to psychic and psychosomatic disturbances. It would be therefore erroneous to make a direct connection between the effect of the thirty-eight Bach Flowers and physical symptoms of illnesses. Bach Flower Therapy is more suited to the field of spiritual health provision.

While Bach Flower Therapy might serve in the prevention of physical illnesses and as a support to a more traditional specialized medical therapy, it should not replace it. When we discuss factors such as diagnosis, patient, therapy, or healing regarding Bach Flower Therapy it should not be interpreted as a prescription. Readers should also understand that Bach Flower Therapy cannot be used in place of treatment by a qualified medical practitioner.

1

HEALING THROUGH THE SOUL

An Introduction to Bach Flower Therapy

When someone is sick he feels and thinks differently. Compared to a healthy person, he may be jittery, resigned, bitter, stubborn, or impatient. As Edward Bach proposed sixty years ago, the patient's consciousness has undergone a negative change by turning away from its higher self and the laws of its soul.* In contrast, a positive change in consciousness— apart from treatments modern medicine might provide—is the deciding factor in every healing process; therefore, every crisis or illness offers us the chance for a positive character change, a step to maturity, a quantum leap in character development.

Edward Bach, among others, observed that with every medically definable illness negative moods such as impatience, despair,

. . . .
* A short overview on the goal of Bach Flower Therapy can be found in appendix one of this book. A detailed description and interpretation of Bach's work is contained in *Bach Flower Therapy*.

and hopelessness become apparent. What is decisive, though, is the fact that every medically definable illness is at some time preceded by such negative moods. If such negative moods can be recognized early on and made positive, physical illness may be prevented altogether.

Today, if one is in a position to take a clear look at our environment, one will notice with horror that a large part of the population of our so-called civilized countries is approaching a state of collective illness. Feelings of resignation, hopelessness, fear, depression, confusion, and helplessness abound and are determining the general feel of life, especially in the younger generation. Perhaps that is why these young people have characteristically been the quickest to recognize and embrace the message of an English physician who combined the abilities of a scientist with those of a modern shaman. Sixty years ago Edward Bach recognized that certain plants have the energetic potency to target negative moods in a subtle way without influencing them arbitrarily. He called them "happy fellows of the plant world," and they served as catalysts for the transformation of negative consciousness into positive consciousness, allowing a profound connection with one's higher self.

Initially viewed with skepticism and the subject of ridicule, Bach Flower Therapy has now become for many people their salvation; it has changed their fate. The following letter from a young Swiss is representative of many others:

> I was born on a farm in Eastern Switzerland, the second of six children. My mother had wished for a girl, but I turned out a boy. Shortly after birth, I developed an eye infection and so I became the problem child of the family. My father tried to break my strong will through punishment and beatings. I had a very hard childhood and I was very defiant. During puberty I often thought of suicide. After school, I worked for a year on the family farm; I was practically

forced to do that. After the year passed, I worked as a letter carrier for the post office. I wanted to get away from the house as soon as possible.

After a year at the post office I got a job with an insurance company. I stayed there for five years. During this time I studied each Saturday in order to obtain a commercial degree. When I was nineteen, I met a man who was thirteen years older and I was drawn to him. My mother was outraged and there were dramatic scenes. But I had my way. Shortly after my departure I also changed jobs. I went to a large bank where I was hired as a computer operator.

The early days with my friend brought many problems. As pressures from home disappeared, many things that had not been dealt with came to the surface. I couldn't manage them by myself. On the advice of my doctor and my friend, I started psychiatric care. My psychiatrist found strong manic-depressive states. He said that it was in my family, that I carried a heavy, hereditary burden. I was on various medications for five years, including Lithium.

For a while I was balanced by the medications. But deep inside of me trouble continued to boil. I started working intensely, as if work was a drug to which I was addicted. I worked at home in the garden, bought animals, half of a farm, all this on top of the work in my office. The drug was outstanding. After fifteen to eighteen hours of work, I would sink into a deep sleep, and all my real problems would seem to move aside. But inside, these pressures took their toll. And so, three years ago, I collapsed and had to be taken to the hospital. I was operated on twice for various cancers, and subsequently underwent twenty sessions of radiation.

My entire outer field of reference—work, the animals, the garden, my friend, my house, my farm—was practically destroyed in one day. I had to give everything up. I only had myself. I was standing in front of nothingness, the ruins of an existence that I had collected for twenty-five years and that I thought represented success. Outwardly and inwardly I was a heap of junk. Negative feelings like hate, envy, jealousy, and many others were determining my being.

By chance I met, at this zero hour, a man who had many times helped his fellow man. I attended his classes and slowly started living again. But because I was still weak and the negative feelings were very strong, I had to pass through the deepest lows once again. Only through the help of my friend was I saved from ruin. Slowly but surely, the climb from the darkness of night into daylight began. In one course I heard something about the Bach Flowers. I was very interested and signed up for an introductory session with great expectations. After a comprehensive discussion, the therapist suggested that I spontaneously pick out six of the thirty-eight small Bach Flower flasks. I pulled out six bottles and was filled with great joy. They were almost all flowers that the therapist had already prescribed in her notes. I had intuitively picked the correct flowers for myself; they were Cerato, Oak, Crab Apple, Wild Oat, Hornbeam, and Willow. I was to take these in four different bottles, in a sequence of four phases.

The first bottle was filled with the Cerato and Oak Bach Flowers. Shortly before I began taking the Bach Flowers, I started working as a gardener for a company that manufactured biological products, cosmetics, and healing aids, among other things. Through my work with the plants in the garden, I experienced a change in myself that was now, by using Cerato and Oak, intensified. I gained great confidence in myself and knew that I was doing the right thing. Through the use of Oak, I stopped looking at my life as a continuing struggle. I started to consciously experience playful and sentimental moments.

I became calm and learned to look at things in a positive light. Living in my new house, working at my new job, I was alone and content. I intentionally wanted to live by myself, in order to cleanse. I wanted to make something positive out of myself, out of my life, before I attempted to live with anybody else again. I was now also free from all medications. I started to expand my consciousness. I read the book *Bach Flower Therapy* and began seeing things as though through different eyes. Finally, after twenty-five years, I started living *my* life. I experienced a great sense of inner joy that filled me almost daily.

The first combination of Cerato/Oak was now replaced by Hornbeam. From this Bach Flower I did not notice anything at first. I tried to gain insight from suggestions in the book. Suddenly I realized that, on a completely different plane, something was starting to stir. I was becoming alive again and started giving in to an unexpected spontaneity. That is something that I have kept to this day: I do what gives me joy, and therefore I remain inwardly and outwardly alive. It was not the outer circumstances that had changed, but so many things were different inwardly that I began to see the world in a new light.

Then it was time for the third phase, Crab Apple and Wild Oat. After all the positive experiences that I had had so far, I learned through the use of Crabapple that no being is completely fulfilled. I understood that something like that was not even possible, otherwise there would be no possibility for learning. I had often had a sensitivity toward, or an obsession for, cleanliness that made me find many things revolting. That now changed. I learned gradually to look at everything from a higher viewpoint, and I saw entirely new connections. Finally I could follow my entire life back to my birth and go through it again, this time from a higher point of view.

And so I started to organize my life anew and brought clarity to all the connections. I was now ready to cleanse not only myself but also the relationships with people from my dark period. I started to accept the scars on my body and realized that the operations had been an opportunity for me. I learned to be grateful for all the learning possibilities my life had given me and started to realize that

I could even help other people through my experiences. Slowly I understood that man has to start at the bottom and climb one step at a time, proving himself worthy with each step he has reached. A rough outline of a goal began to take shape, a goal that had always slumbered deep inside of me. In order to achieve this goal, I had many steps to take. The energy of the Wild Oat gave me the leading thread or direction to achieve the goal.

It was at this time that I met my future wife. I immediately had the certitude that she was the right one. We married shortly after our first meeting. To this day I have never regretted that step; I also have the certainty that I never will.

The final Bach Flower that closes this therapy is Willow. Through Willow I learned to take responsibility for my destiny. I recognized that everything that happened was ultimately due to what I was carrying inside of me. I now know that the darkness in my life has given me a great opportunity for learning. Was I not the builder of my own destiny? I had arranged the stones in my quarry, so that now I could build a house with them. It was not the bad disease or evil doctor who had given me all this suffering, all the scars. No, I alone was the perpetrator and the victim. All the things that I did to myself finally allowed me to reach a point where I could be rational and could courageously view problems as chances to learn. I try now to do justice to the lesson I've learned.

The Bach Flowers were catalysts for me. They gave me the strength and courage to see myself as I really am, and to be able to say yes to myself. They haven't changed anything about me externally and yet they have changed everything. They have helped to merge my body, soul, and spirit, have given them the opportunity to work together. Two drops out of a thirty-milliliter bottle of water and alcohol. No scientific thinker will accept that! The Bach Flowers help one find the way inward. Often one must clear the blocked street or shovel the snowed-in road. It takes longer to reach one's goal, but once the road is free and clear, we are free to travel it, with all its consequences; this road is always worth it.

The positive restructuring of one's personality is not always experienced as dramatically as in the previous account. Often, the positive transformation of one's consciousness is initially apparent only in smaller, seemingly trivial behavioral changes. A fifty-year-old consultant from an old military family wrote:

> The first time I had a very positive experience. My furrier promised to do an alteration for me at a low summer price—"maybe it will cost fifty marks," he had said. When I went to pick up the alteration with a friend, the furrier himself was not there. His mother handed me a bill that was 100 marks higher, because supposedly new fur had to be used. I left it at that, which was a pattern of mine—always putting up with this type of situation. A couple of days later it suddenly hit me. I got on the phone, spoke to the furrier right away and explained my situation to him. He explained it as an error on the part of his mother, and said I should deduct the 100 marks from the final bill. It was that simple! For the first time I had consciously stood for what was rightfully mine. For me that was an experience.

In some cases, new perspectives and realizations for the spiritual and soulful development of the personality are obtained after a relatively short period of treatment. A Swiss social worker writes, "In my religious development I experienced a positive step in the direction of faith, trust, and the ability to pray without making any special effort."

In every case one can conclude that Bach Flower Therapy sets in motion a positive process of development. According to one psychologist: "The question, if the problem of a personal situation has been solved, cannot always be answered unequivocally. But the development process has been set in motion, and has such an indi-vidual course, that it sometimes cannot be verbalized for other people."

Following is a typical account after therapy of a few weeks, in which the author, a naturopath, has been participating in a seminar:

Today is the end of the first bottle, and with it the first cycle of my drops. What I have learned so far with their help is, I think, the ability to touch my own shadows. I studied many things outwardly that I thought could never be inside of me, because they made me feel so uncomfortable and ashamed. But obviously these feelings are part of me.

Aggression, fear, hate, and despair all lived deeply hidden in my inner self and suddenly, with the use of drops, I experienced them outwardly for the first time. Things were happening to me that, I am certain, would have never occurred if I had not been ready for them. I fear that I have experienced and discovered only a very small part of my shadowy side, but I believe very strongly that my body and my soul will only let me deal with as much as I can handle. Some-how, this thought gives me confidence in myself and I feel protected and sheltered.

2

WHAT IS THE COURSE
of a Bach Flower Therapy?

Because Bach Flower Therapy corresponds to the inner powers of each individual, we can safely say that there are no two identical developments resulting from the same Bach Flower Therapy. With a Bach Flower Therapy it does not make much sense to try to develop either a course of action or a record of symptoms as one might in a true homeopathic repertoire. Trying to do so would shift one's view from what is best and unique about Bach Flower Therapy, which is the inner dynamic of the individual.

The course of therapy depends on a constellation of occurrences, which takes into account both the history of the patients and their surroundings, but above all the "quality of time." All of these factors play a deciding role and color patients' symptoms in an individual fashion. Because these factors are unique to a given moment and person, the development and course of a therapy cannot be repeated.

While the observations presented here are drawn from twelve years of practice with Bach Flowers, they may serve to inspire awareness of the beginning Bach Flower patient's own observations.

Primary reactions that could appear in the first days after starting the therapy include:

a. A deep inhalation and a change in eye expression immediately after ingestion
b. Intensified sensory perception
c. Feelings of warmth and joy throughout the entire body
d. Reactions, as if responding to sensations caused by electricity, a sting, a flash, a prickly feeling, cold, etc., especially on the left side of the body
e. A strong need for rest or sleep because so much energy is being used up on an inner plane
f. A sense of dizziness or confusion during the day
g. A metallic taste in the mouth
h. Flashes of past-disease symptoms, such as rheumatic aches or pains
i. An outer sign of psychic cleansing in the form of rashes that subside in two to three days—for example, eczema on the left hand, an outbreak on the skin of the right index and ring fingers, or strong itching on the heels, knees, and elbows
j. Heavy menstrual flow in women
k. Dreams about keys during the first night

The following passage describes the appearance of immediate reactions with subsequent physical symptoms after taking a mixture of Heather, Holly, and Pine.

I took the first four drops in the evening around seven o'clock. Later, between ten and eleven o'clock, I was going to bed and was standing in my bathroom when I let out a groan. I was very astonished, especially since it was followed by similar outbursts—moans and groans and then whimpering that changed to crying. The words came to me: flayed creature. All this seemed to come from a place over which I had no influence. I was bewildered and felt like a spectator. In the night I had an attack of angina that I had felt coming on a little in the evening. It was very strong, a feeling I hadn't experienced in years.

In the next few days—I had a lot of time to myself, but somehow I couldn't rest—in front of my eyes there appeared a kind of fog bank that parted. Then I saw two layers of fog. One layer below, on the ground, and a vague second layer above it, with imperceptible shapes in it of about one meter in height.

My angina and the sniffles, combined with the feeling that something was happening inside me, gave me peace, and I appreciated the opportunity of being able to be alone without having to be constantly busy.

After about four or five days it was clear that something massive—something that had built up inside of me—began to break up. I felt like I was standing slightly to the side but at the same time was more connected with myself.

A second example of an immediate reaction after taking Hornbeam:

I had planned this morning to ride my bicycle to town on a few important errands. Suddenly I felt like I was nailed to my kitchen chair; I was overwhelmed by exhaustion and a melancholic state of mind. My first thoughts were that I should sell my practice and that nothing works anymore. What was happening? Were these the first signs of an illness coming on? Forcibly, I pulled myself together and took my bicycle out of the garage. I had to somehow be able to do this. After riding for about 400 meters (luckily I was still on side streets), there was a powerful twitch in my left arm as if I had been electrocuted. It scared me and I could hardly keep the bicycle under control. Should I continue? I did, but not for long. The same convulsive jerk now happened in my right thigh! Only then did it occur to me that this could be a reaction to the Bach Flowers.

Then I was calm. Nothing else exciting happened. Around two o'clock in the afternoon I felt a distinct stabilization and strengthening of my energy. It was a wonderful adventure.

Another patient describes an intensification of consciousness that sometimes occurs in reaction to the Bach Flower Remedies: "I was listening to Piano Concertos numbers three and five by Beethoven with Alfred Brendel. An entirely new musical experience. The music was overwhelming. Huge rooms were opening up in which the notes were moving around . . ."

In the next two examples, we see the experiences of an inner joy and a feeling of wellness that sets in after taking the Bach Flowers:

It is nine o'clock in the evening, one hour after my first dose. My husband, who doesn't know anything about my therapy, says, "You speak differently; you are so quiet!" I can't see the change myself. At 9:30 I go to bed.

I am alone. Peace. Peace flows through my arms and hands. I am quiet and as clear as a mountain lake. From the deep, a fine, delicate but perceptible stream rises to, and above, the surface (my body). It has a goal. Does it turn to those maternal beings that unselfishly offer us their flowing flowers? What is it? A giving? A taking? A loving, wordless dialogue? A linked compromise? How little I know about my soul. God, open my eyes!

I would like to describe briefly the first reaction that I experienced with Agrimony. A half hour after I took the essence I felt uplifted. A feeling of joy rose in me. I felt elevated and happy. I had a fit of laughter that lasted fifteen minutes. After that the feelings were a little subdued, but for the rest of the day I felt bright and cheerful.

A typical example of having multiple primary reactions after taking a combination of Crab Apple, Cerato, Vervain, and Olive, as related by one seminar participant:

Primary reactions: After six days of intake—tiredness and the feeling something is at work around the kidneys. Many dreams—for the most part very recognizable. I can understand them. I need a lot of sleep. A lot of energy flowing through my legs, a strong downward pull.

Developments: Loss of concentration, fatigue, the right side of my body feels blocked. After three days things get better.

Status: Deep breathing, a feeling of ease, a clear head and, especially, eyes. The feeling of energy flowing through my entire body. Many dreams.

Powerful dreams are very typical on the first night after intake. They reveal the many ways in which the structure of the unconscious has been set in a positive motion.

A twenty-four-year-old patient, who in the past had smoked a lot and on occasion used drugs recreationally, experienced in her second night of therapy a warning from her inner doctor: "A face of someone I know well, wearing a white frock, listens to my smoker's cough. He examines me and says that if I continue smoking, in a year I will cough blood." Often, the unconscious will signal when a growing process is being introduced, as described by the following patients. After using Walnut and Elm, a dancer reports: "I have powerful impressive dreams. The messages are often simple (once I was a switch-man at a railway station). After three days of therapy I feel very clear and relaxed." A student nurse tells us: "I was riding my bicycle on a leaf-covered road. I was wondering why the road was so dark and the lights on my bicycle were very weak. I knew that in order to continue along this road I would need a lot of strength to pedal. Then I woke up."

One seminar participant from Vienna, after taking Gentian: "There is a bathtub in this strange house. I take a bath. As I get out of the tub, I put on a bathrobe. I feel well and rejuvenated. In my right hand I have a container. It holds many blue bath crystals. As I leave the bathroom, the house opens up into a huge landscape." The bath here is seen as a symbol of change and cleansing. The water symbolizes the psychic energy that is in this case being absorbed by the dreamer. A similar symbol of cleansing is snow, as in the following dream description: "I am driving my car. A powerful snowstorm begins . . ."

One symbolic dreamscape of a forty-five-year-old patient points to the development of an internal process: "I brush my teeth thoroughly, until they bleed." In this case the teeth symbolize strength, vitality, and, in certain situations, aggression.

A fifty-eight-year-old female has a dream involving blood and writes: "The second night, I dreamt that I got a very strong menstrual period." Dreams of this sort are frequent and very interesting. If one considers blood as representing the seat of the soul and as a symbol of the life force, one can view dreams in which bleeding occurs as suggestive of renewal and fruitfulness, and as involving a fecundity of psychic activity.

Indicative of the fact that the new growing processes of the Higher Self are being gladly accepted and greeted are dreams such as:

In the middle of a very tiring bicycle ride on a long, dusty, and endless road, I suddenly stopped and got off the bicycle. I found myself below a huge rosebush and I started to pick the life-bestowing flowers for myself and put them in my backpack for the return trip.

The roses here are also to be understood as symbols of fruitfulness and of godly love.

A client writes, "My therapist is teaching me how to play the piano and at the end of the lesson she hands me a little white lamb. My feelings during the dream are those of a small child." Playing the piano symbolizes the school of life, and the lamb—according to Christian symbolism (contrast of lion to lamb)—the sign of a human being who is in complete control of his strengths and powers.

In another group of dreams it appears that previously repressed or unrecognized psychic details come to the forefront and connect with other levels of consciousness: A doctor dreams, "The moon winked at me, closed both eyes, and opened them up again."

A student writes, "I was bathing in a crystal-clear lake in the middle of a large landscape." A fifty-two-year-old widow's account: "I went to a wedding. There were a lot of people there, all from my youth, from my school days. I was supposed to sing with a group, and I was uncertain about my voice, but I didn't have to sing the lead. We all wanted to sing. Heaven and Earth must pass by, but the music stays constant." The wedding is to be interpreted as a symbol of the union of the spirit and soul with the physical body.

On the second day of Flower intake, a naturopath recounted the following from two dreams: "I met somebody I cared about. He apologized for not keeping in touch," and "I had a small child again that I cared for and loved."

Other dreams symbolize the struggle between the new constructive powers and the entrenched, underlying, negative states.

I am being threatened by a powerful, angry man. I feel too weak to be able to withstand any of this primordial violence. I can only shy away. Later in the dream my powers have grown, and I can imagine punching him in the nose. Are these my own primordial forces that at first scared me but which I learned how to live with and control?

. .

I sat in a car with a man who wanted to take my precious chess pieces away from me. I store them in four white boxes, just like the Bach Flower essences. Just as the man appeared triumphant, seeing that I had them with me, I noticed that I was sitting on them. I grabbed the boxes, jumped out of the car and ran into a forest. I could not run as fast as I wanted to, and I knew that I would eventually get caught, but at the same time I knew everything would be all right.

The image of the chess pieces is an interesting one. In this example it symbolizes the dreamer's ability to play the game of life.

A fifty-two-year-old painter dreams: "I am walking in the woods when suddenly a barking deer runs toward me. I'm afraid that it's rabid and wants to bite me. I tell it to sit. The deer listens and doesn't move from its spot as I go on my way. I am no longer afraid."

The deer is also a symbol of the soul. It embodies the feminine and earthen sides inherent in the duality of sky and earth. The dream may suggest how the patient initially seemed fearful of these Flowers that seemed at first uncontrollable (symbolized by the rabid deer), but in the end the Flowers are consciously controllable. The same patient later had two more dreams that make the progress of the therapy clear. First, she reports, "I am lowering heavy metal balls, that are tied with a ribbon, into a well, and then I am cutting the ribbon." Subsequently, she confronts a new crisis, which she quickly overcomes:

I dream that a heavy, overloaded truck drives out of the water and onto a street. The driver has to make a turn and backs the truck onto a street that is high above the water, without any railings. With my heart beating fast, I see the truck rolling toward the edge of the precipice, but the driver manages to stop the truck a few centimeters before the edge. The load on the truck sways back and forth, but it doesn't fall. When I wake up, my heart is beating very strongly.

COURSE OF DEVELOPMENT

These are experiences from many years of a Bach Flower Therapy practice and they shouldn't be looked upon as absolute rules, but, especially for beginners, as helpful suggestions.

Depending on the starting point and inner goals one sets for the therapy, there are distinct courses of development to be seen.

Situation 1:

An acute negative state is being treated. For example:

I have a lot of work to do, which leaves little time for reading, except at night; undisturbed, I try to concentrate and study. But I get overwrought. My head hurts, thoughts buzz around, and I lose all strength. My eyes water. . . . I reach for Hornbeam and rub a drop straight from the bottle on my forehead, eyes, and neck. Then I sleep long and deep and wake up refreshed! My head is clear and my eyes are no longer watering.

. .

After a hectic day I get home exhausted and I am burdened with haunting images that I would like to get rid of. I put three drops each of Crab Apple and Olive into my bathwater. That same evening I have a tranquil feeling, a feeling of being myself again.

. .

I have to do my homework, but its subject matter doesn't particularly interest me. My thoughts drift constantly to situations that are closer to my heart, like planning next spring's garden. I put two drops of Clematis into a glass of water and drink the entire glass over the course of the day. The next day I have my thoughts fully on my work.

In an acute state, the use of the correct Bach Flowers can have a positive effect in a few hours or, in some cases, a few days.

Situation 2:

A chronic condition is being treated. In this kind of a situation character traits are always involved, depending on age and living situation, that undergo slow changes of structure under the influence of tenacious inner struggles. Depending on an individual's inner development phase, the therapy can require weeks, months, or as much as two years to take effect. Example: A married woman is in a dependent relationship with her mother-in-law, is always afraid for her kids, and suffers for many years from various neuro-vegetative disturbances. In chronic situations such as this, a high percentage of the cases fall into one of two categories of reaction possibilities.

CATEGORY 1
For a few weeks, the Bach Flowers have a surprisingly positive effect. The initial reaction is mainly "I haven't felt this good in many

years." After a few weeks the curve may fall off, and then the patient experiences the ups and downs of her own psychic and physical states, which eventually will stabilize toward the positive, as shown in the graph below.

Category 1

Patient's
development

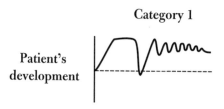

The Flower combination for this first positive phase was appropriately named by a patient "mercy flowers." Only after the second up-and-down cycle will an inner peace and one's own weaknesses of character become part of the growing process. A patient describes this vividly:

We were in agreement that man has a certain grace period in which the flowers work without his help. After that one has to work very hard *with* them. When people say that suddenly the flowers don't seem to help anymore they should examine the reason for that.

Since the flowers affect all the changes in us, it is important to register and work with these changes. This manner of cooperation allowed me, with each new recipe from the book, to follow through and try to learn about blocked and hidden emotions. It is important to accept them. Afterward, though, I concentrated on only the transformed states and imagined these full of life. I lived that way, through altering my thoughts. It is not a new idea that one can change who one is by transforming how one thinks. There is a saying, "A steady drop will make a hole in the stone." When, at each intake of the Flower essences, I visualize the transformed states, that is already cooperation. I have conducted myself in this fashion during the two years of my flower therapy and I see a lot of progress in myself.

The Bach Flowers exist to help you help yourself.

CATEGORY 2

The patient experiences a very powerful psychic and/or physical intensification of symptoms, similar to a primary, homeopathic reaction. This state can last for days or, in an extreme situation, for weeks, after which it will abruptly improve. With this time frame we also see the up-and-down cycles that will eventually stabilize on a higher level.

Category 2

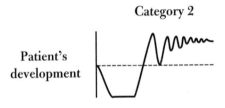

Patient's development

During that first phase, the patient will be quite beside himself and may call his practitioner many times, quite terrified, and say, "I haven't felt this terrible in years." And then suddenly one day things will go decisively better.

In a low state such as the aforementioned one the patient can augment his therapy by taking emergency drops. It is recommended to reduce the normal dose of four drops four times daily, to three drops three times daily or two drops two times daily.

In such situations it is important to know that the accentuated negative feelings and symptoms are just expressions of the spiritual and psychic cleansing processes, without which the step to true healing cannot be taken.

As one patient spontaneously realized in conversation, "In my opinion, the flowers bring a deficient circumstance clearly into your consciousness before it disappears." And as a seminar participant writes:

> In principle, I've always made the same discovery; what was so agonizing had until that time been very successfully repressed and was only brought into consciousness by the drops. It may involve emotions or needs that were never satisfied—rage, or hate, or anger. It makes no difference. . . .

There are cases where, for some people, the accentuation of symptoms will appear again, albeit in a weaker form, after repeated intake of a flower combination. On the other hand, there are others who, during the entire duration of their therapy, may never experience intense symptom accentuation. A Swiss lady writes, "What amazes me is that I never experienced any intensification of symptoms, or at least I didn't recognize them. But I always strongly felt the change that was happening on a psychic plane."

What is important in this second category is to continue the therapy. It would be a mistake to interrupt the therapy at the appearance of the first negative reaction, only to try it again later. The only thing an interruption would accomplish is a delay in the healing process. Here is a typical case reported by a Swiss healer:

> A sixteen-year-old patient who had always been suspicious of the therapy reported that he had started wetting his bed after intake. He stopped the therapy and the occurrences stopped also. After a while he started the therapy again, and became a bed wetter again. This time he stopped the program permanently. If, after the first interruption, he could have worked on the psychic background of his bed-wetting (daily consciousness, repressed fear, an inability to

cry), it is presumable that he would have made it through the second time around, and his bed-wetting would have disappeared.

It has often been observed that during a Bach Flower Therapy many patients are able to gradually discontinue their use of psychotropic drugs. In rare cases, even after making great mental progress with the Bach Flowers, a dependency on the addictive psychotropic drugs is still present, albeit in very reduced form. In this sort of an emergency one can take such a drug in the smallest of doses.

The following is a list of typical positive reactions that can appear after a long-term therapy with the Bach Flowers:

a. Facial expressions are softened; psychic outlook is markedly positive.

b. Changes will be perceived by others, even before the patient notices: "One can talk to you again."

c. The patient looks visibly younger, almost childlike: "Recently I was mistaken for the daughter of a colleague who is my age."

d. The patient can cry again.

e. Emotional states are being consciously experienced once again. One can distance oneself from the actual occurrence: "It seemed as if I was standing next to it."

f. An inclination to clarify things increases. (Often, environmental factors will bring about clarification.)

g. Sensory experiences are heightened. The patient can hear better, see better, smell again: "I smelled a blossoming field of wheat, and started crying for joy!"

h. Physiological change is magnified, such as loss of excess weight; the digestive system works better; there is better circulation in the hands and feet; skin disorders and headaches disappear.

i. The patient develops a sensitivity to alcohol.

j. Other treatments improve as well. For example, breathing therapists, massage therapists, and music teachers notice the differences in their patient or student. For the music teacher: "I noticed, with astonishment, that the voice had become fuller and more powerful."

k. Dreaming becomes more vivid; dreams are more colorful. After some time, many childhood dreams recur.

Respective to point j, a patient writes:

"After a few weeks of the Bach flowers, I noticed that the problems I had with my arms and hands were greatly improved. After a two-week break, my naturopath noticed during a lymph-draining procedure that "everything has become amazingly free." That was confirmation for me: "Flowers that heal through the soul."

Following are descriptions of two dreams that signal the successful completion of a Bach Flower Therapy:

I lie on my back and look up at a green canopy. There is an image in a round frame. Right above me are two large hands that are being held out to me. I know that God is offering me his help, and that he will pull me up if I grab his hands, and that he will stand me up on my feet.

· ·

It is as if I am waking up. On my left there are two little girls. I recognize the one to the right; she is about five years old and very pale, delicate and loving. It seems as though there is no blood running through her. She gives me a kiss on the forehead and I wake up with a good, promising feeling.

One seminar participant's comprehensive report contains many details characteristic of Bach Flower Therapy and emphasizes the importance of individuality in responding to the Flower Remedies:

> The therapy will work mainly on things that are largely unknown to us and on untransformed layers of consciousness, and is therefore a wonderful help in the sense of "Become what you are and you will know it."
>
> The perception of the effects occurs mainly on a plane involving feelings related to inner experiences. After the intake of my flower combinations, everything became clearer. I realize daily how I become more aware of various layers of my whole self. My entire being becomes individualized in its view of origin and goal. At intake, as well as during any activity involving the Bach Flowers, I often feel deep gratitude for this gift, and the feeling of love I have for all beings and plants becomes stronger.
>
> The Bach Remedies are giving me an increased understanding of the different traits and characteristics of being, of man. From that comes the development of tolerance and the possibility of accepting all beings as individuals. The physical healing is almost a by-product of the inner healing; in other words, the work affects us from the inside out.
>
> Physically, I feel the effects of the Bach Flowers working in certain areas, specifically in past-disease areas—on pain from old scar tissue, or where headaches were very frequent. For a time my hair would literally stand up. Was that a sign of active work inside my head? Healing on my entire body was felt as a cleansing phase. Sometimes I can almost predict which particular flower in the combination works at a certain time and when it releases its healing powers.
>
> What impresses me the most is that the Flower Therapy works in such a clear, simple way, without encroaching into the psychic

organism of man in any "unnatural" manner. The flowers can only inspire a spiritual and psychic development process; they cannot enforce it. Each individual therefore has a hand in the extent of the effects, and has to earn them inwardly.

3

THE BACH FLOWERS

as *Developmental Aids in the Ordering of Oneself*

Edward Bach perceived that his flowers would ultimately be present in
every household. Amazing is
the degree with which his
message has influenced the
circles of those who are
spiritually open-minded. The enthusiasm
for the idea of "healing through the soul"
transcends all population and age groups. It
reaches from the sixteen-year-old student to the
seventy-six-year-old advanced-education advisers, from the hair-
dresser to the psychology professor to the opera singer. Those
whose work requires that they lead and advise others have discovered
the Bach Flowers. The esoterically inclined use them for the support of
their self-developmental work. In particular, many mothers use the Bach
Flowers as a blessing for themselves and their families.

The question of determining the most suitable Bach Flower
combination can be solved quite unproblematically in these cases. We
are dealing here with psychologically healthy people, of well-known

character. Therefore the respective spiritual state can be easily established with knowledge and research of individual flower descriptions.

An additional aid, especially when making a selection for older members of one's family, for small children, or for one's self, has proven to be the "grab test," in which intuition comes to the forefront. This sort of random diagnosis may appear illogical to a scientifically minded person, but it has proven itself in practice thousands of times. As a nurse from Austria writes:

> I lay all 38 Bach Flower essence bottles on the table. Then quickly, one after the other, without any wishful thinking or expectations, I pick six of them. Afterward, when I read the descriptions of the psychological states that each flower corresponds to, and bring them into the context of my own character and present situation, it turns out that for this time frame I have selected the correct flowers 60–90 percent of the time. Many of the flowers I might never have tried, had I relied on a purely intellectual self-analysis. The only possible explanation of this phenomenon is that in this spontaneous, quick grabbing, either the Higher Self or the inner doctor is being activated, without being blocked by reasoning or doubt.

A naturopath adds to this theme:

> Certain essences that were initially considered to be picked in error turn out to have a meaningful selection. With Cherry Plum the shock came after two days, whereas Mustard, picked in the best of psychic states, turned out to be, two days later, very necessary. (In both cases I did not use them in the mixture and learned later, in hindsight, that the soul knew better than the head.)
>
> A friend grabbed Scleranthus from among some others and protested that she didn't need this essence, because she was not in a situation where she would have to make any important decisions.

Three days later, out of the blue, she had to decide whether to separate from her boyfriend. Other self-pickers confirm the fact that the flowers indicated feelings or situations they had already sensed, dreamed about, or envisioned.

This declaration should not lead to misuse or to viewing the Bach Flowers as either an I Ching replacement or an oracle in liquid flower form which some might be tempted to do in their initial excitement. Those spiritually interested or holistically inclined have the tendency to lose, in certain phases of their development, the realistic outlook of the connection between soul, body, and spirit. For them there is the advice of an esoterically well-informed Swiss healer:

The designation "holistic" is being played with a lot these days. Where one talks about spirit, soul, and body, one constantly refers to the "fine matter." Before one evaluates the "fine matter" one should connect it to the "coarse matter." The "coarse matter" or physical body is subject to the physical rules in the name of God. (These can be disturbed through one's psyche.) The fact that the human machine has to be cared for and kept in tune just like a vehicle is something that many "spirit seekers" are missing. A weak body with an ineffective metabolism is not very helpful when one demands "fine matter" development.

The physical body has certain energy connections which create zones between the fine and the coarse matter. The nerves play an important role in this system; but in order to have the energies work together well in the coarse matter, one has to make sure the "wiring" is correct and functional.

At this point it should be noted that the essence of Rock Water can be helpful in bringing the interdependent relationships of soul, spirit, and body back into consciousness.

Personal and Self-therapies in General Human Crises

Weak will due to overdemand—
personal experience with Centaury.

My son, who is twenty-two years old, comes home for a few days. I feel tired and run down; I feel weight on my shoulders. Nothing really matters.

The second day one of my son's comments rattles me. He can see through the situation: "What is happening to you? You seem to let everything just go by. You can't even say 'no' anymore!". . . I pull back. He's right. I am imagining the result of my behavior, especially in regards to my youngest, who is ten years old. I have to change it. But how? I ask for inner guidance.

The next day during some housecleaning I notice the book Bach Flower Therapy. *I grab it, leave everything else, and start leafing through it. Centaury is it! I know it suddenly.*

I set up my bottle as directed; first dose before lunch, second one before bedtime.

I am calm, quiet, and relaxed. I feel as if the petals of a large flower have closed over my head, just as some flowers do before bad weather; it's as if a deep wound on my left side is healing. . . . I sleep calmly and deeply. After I wake, I have the need to stretch out and straighten up. I feel as if I've grown a few centimeters. . . . I visibly gain energy and strength.

After a few days, I feel as I did in my younger years; I have the desire to do things and my youngest can't get away with everything anymore. After a week, I forget about the dosage. I don't need Centaury anymore.

A medical student discovers
the needy child in herself

If anybody, anywhere has ever fit the image of Heather, then that was me, at least until the time that I started meditating. Until then,

I could never keep my mouth shut. I would talk on and on.

I must have been quite a scary sight to other people, because I never gave them the opportunity to interrupt me. In school I felt like I should always have the last word! I used to cry and be insulting when I wasn't included in conversations. In my circle of friends I thought I was loved, because I was always cheerful, joked a lot, and gravitated toward somebody if I saw that they were alone.

I needed these discussions, especially my participation in them, in order to prove to myself that there was nothing wrong with me, because earlier I had never really had true friends. I had never belonged to a clique. I avoided people but at the same time I needed them. And when somebody would tell me that I had no idea what I was talking about, I felt shocked and discouraged. I wanted to pretend that I was clever and intelligent, but in reality I was stupid and ignorant. I realized that those who criticized my chatter were right, and yet I still could not do anything about my ignorance; therefore I felt more compelled to talk and at the same time despised myself. As I started to meditate and new thoughts appeared, I lost the need to talk about everything, and for the first time my life had a purpose that I followed with joy and zeal. But it wasn't hard to realize that the Heather problem could not have disappeared so easily; it had just taken an introverted form: I seldom spoke and tried to figure everything out in my thoughts. My relatives realized right away that I wasn't talking anymore. But what should I talk about? I didn't know anything that was true.

For years now, on my summer vacations, I have been going to a camp where I am among like-minded people. There we have daily discussion sessions. It was here that my Heather state expressed itself the most. I would painfully search for questions and contributions to share, which often resulted in embarrassing situations or answers to my questions that made me look stupid. As much as I wished to be able to be quiet, to just listen and think like everybody else, I couldn't help myself. I needed confirmation that I had worth and thought that it would happen through people paying attention to me and praising my contributions. At some point somebody had to tell me to my face that I was being disruptive (this was the opposite of what I had in mind). That is when I picked up Heather.

Before long I began carrying the stock bottle around with me and felt like I was becoming calmer inwardly. Then I started taking the drops on a regular basis and noticed a reduced need to speak. At the same time I became more aware of why I so painfully sought out people and conversations. It was as if I wore a tight dress that finally ripped open and I started getting more air. I felt, after a long time, at home in my own body. That was the beginning. As time went by, it became easier to listen, to be quiet. My problem wasn't completely solved through Heather, but I had broken through to the next layer.

Reanimation and uplifting personal experience with Star of Bethlehem

On April 9, 1982, I took Star of Bethlehem for the first time. That same night I had intense dreams and entered a dream phase that lasted a few weeks. I often remembered details in the morning. Most dreams were very archaic and dealt with childhood or very early childhood—before the birth of my brother. I recalled scenes from an apartment where we lived until I was about four years old and shocking situations that I had lived through. On occasion I vividly remembered people with whom I hadn't been in contact for more than fifteen years. I encountered situations that I remember myself being in, but in the similar situations I reacted in a completely opposite and negative manner. As I was experiencing smaller and greater disappointments, I remember here and there how I had myself been guilty of similar actions toward other people.

I have an almost personal relationship with Star of Bethlehem. I buy this flower very often. Once, in the summer of 1983, I found a large collection of them in a field. I dug one up and planted it on my terrace. Quite early on the leaves began to sprout. This plant has brought me a lot of joy.

A mother provides therapy for her son

Andreas grew up as an only child, with no friends or play-mates. He stayed busy by himself, loved to build things, and was very creative. He was very timid and found it difficult to make contact with people.

His first two years of school were a catastrophe. Within the first three weeks all of his creativity had disappeared. He made no contact with other children and things were stolen from him. . . . He withdrew completely. His teacher seemed interested only in his studies. Behaviors of his that did not fall within the realm of her teaching methods received no attention. Andreas became stubborn, purposely gave wrong answers, was restless, and became aggressive. He was labeled as anti-social.

With a lot of love and patience I managed to turn him around. The next two school years went by more favorably. His new teacher dealt with him without prejudice. Still, it took over a year for Andreas to win his confidence back, to willingly do his homework, and to answer his teacher's questions in an audible voice.

I dared to enroll Andreas in a middle school because one teacher remarked that he might not be challenged enough. We still had reservations about his social behavior.

During his summer holidays in August, I chose two flowers for him, Holly and Mimulus, based on Bach Flower Therapy. *He was already getting Rescue Remedy in cream form rubbed onto his forehead; he never would take any other sort of medicine in situations where he was getting very worked up or aggressive. Now and then, he started asking for the cream himself.*

Three days after taking Holly and Mimulus, Andreas became more cheerful. He was looser, more relaxed, and laughed out loud, even about his own fits of rage! After a week he showed interest in new games, started joking around, and for the first time went on a bicycle trip with his classmates.

Three days before school started I gave him a combination recommended in Bach Flower Therapy *for the time when school begins, as well as continuing with Holly and Mimulus. The transition to school went quite smoothly. Andreas got out of bed as soon as he woke up (which was never the case in primary school), did his homework right after lunch without being asked, and seemed content. Since hardly anybody can get off a beaten track on the first try, starting October second I gave him Mimulus, Chestnut Bud, Impatiens, Holly, and Aspen. Andreas willingly took his drops on schedule.*

Middle of October: consulting with his teachers, I heard of no further problems; he seemed to be a little unfocused, but he asked his teacher questions and at times thought ahead.

October 16: I replaced Holly with Willow because Andreas became very selfish. Aspen fell by the wayside.

Nov. 5: Andreas didn't study because he thought everything would be as easy as primary school. He was tired, had trouble falling asleep, and had headaches. He got some bad grades. The strain of waking up at 5:45 A.M. and coming home from school at 2 P.M. was noticeable. I gave him Clematis, Willow, Gentian, White Chestnut. He had to go to bed earlier!

Result: Andreas's grades improved dramatically. He went to school willingly and showed interest. After the bottle was nearly empty, we forgot about the drops.

December 12: Andreas's eyes were puffy and he had dark rings around them. He didn't eat; he seemed beaten down and crushed. He went quietly to bed and I rubbed some Rescue Remedy on his forehead.

December 13: Our naturopath diagnosed a cold and a bad kidney function. Andreas took homeopathic drops. He didn't want to open up to me. I had the feeling he was keeping something inside, but I didn't want to pressure him to tell me.

December 14: Andreas got Mimulus, Olive, Gorse, Chestnut Bud, Gentian, and Larch.

December 17: My son, although he seemed healthy, didn't want to go to school anymore. He failed an exam. He got Rescue Remedy on his forehead again and I promised not to wake him the next day; he could sleep in and then we could talk about it.

December 19: Andreas went back to school.

December 20: A reprimand arrived home from school for December 12. With hesitation Andreas told me the truth. At the end of the second period, as the teacher was correcting some papers, he took a bite out of his sandwich. When the teacher asked him what he was doing, he put his sandwich away and said "nothing." For that a reprimand! Some time away from school, and my speaking out against such treatment, has put everything back in order.

Today, Andreas gladly goes to school. His grades are pretty good. His report card notes that his work is worthy of acknowledgement and his behavior is adequate. We are all satisfied.

How many children who are tired of school and are sulky and listless could be helped in this manner? How many could avoid being sent to special education schools?

A problem that appears in every relationship

My husband gets his way more often and more easily than I do. After the last time we made love—an enormous effort on my part since I was very tired—I had the feeling that I shouldn't have said yes. For days I felt tired, had pain in my pelvis, and felt confused and troubled over issues of absolute spiritual closeness.

I have to learn not to say yes, just because I fear his anger. Claus will have to learn, just like me. I get depressed when he turns away. He has childish reactions, and I'm hurt by his reproach—"he might have to make an appointment with me." He doesn't realize how his demeanor drains me.

Love for me is most of all a spiritual union, one that is only expressed physically secondarily. He looks for the same thing, only in a man's way. When he is gentle and delicate toward me, everything is different. Only rarely do we have discussions about feelings or daily concerns. I will take more Heather, in order to be able to listen better. And Centaury will help me to not subjugate myself to his demands anymore.

An Austrian Bach Flower user
helps his relatives

This has to do with my sister and her family from Geneva. My sister, Mrs. Gerti F., is forty-three years old, a housewife, Austrian by birth. Since the death of our mother in 1967, my sister has had a terrible fear of cancer. She constantly feared for her two sons, Daniel (19) and Michael (21), as well as for her husband. She would go twice a year for a mammography and would send her relatives to the doctor constantly. In addition she was always very nervous and tense.

In August of 1982 my sister came to Vienna for a holiday, and I talked to her about the Bach Flowers. I made a mixture for her of Mimulus, Aspen, and Star of Bethlehem. I also gave her Vervain since she sometimes went overboard by trying too hard. She took these drops for almost a year. When she surprised us with a visit in November of 1982 she told us one evening: "I have no fear of cancer anymore; I feel well. We even go out every week now."

My brother-in-law, Gerd F., forty-four years old, an officer at a bank and a Swiss citizen, told me a few times how he felt worthless because he had masturbated a few times in his youth. He felt full of guilt. He was a Wild Rose type because he was not much of a participant. Sometimes he wouldn't utter more than ten short sentences a week, and lately he didn't want to be among people anymore. I advised a mixture of Pine and Star of Bethlehem and continued with a combination of Wild Rose, Crab Apple, and Centaury—the last one because he would never utter an opinion about anything.

By November, he too was unrecognizable—relaxed, cheerful, and talkative like never before. He said, "Things are going very well for me now."

4
EXPERIENCES
with Animals and Plants

There are many reports of treating animals and plants* with Bach Flower Remedies, especially with Rescue Remedy.

Many people ask if animals, who don't have an individuality comparable to humans, can get any help from the Bach Flowers. Our experience so far has shown that treating symptoms of animals in an acute state can lead to amazingly quick recovery. Animals in a chronic state who found help from Bach Flowers were seen to have all their symptoms return as soon as the treatment was stopped. For example, an old, epileptic fox terrier was treated with Mimulus on a regular basis. As the therapy was discontinued, the attacks started again. Reintroducing Mimulus stopped them again.

. . . .
* The dosage used for treating animals and plants has not been established exactly and is left to intuition. Suggestion based on experience: four drops from a stock bottle per bowl, or ten drops for a ten-liter bucket.

It is easy to imagine that animals might benefit from the same plants that the owner is using, or from plants with which the owner has a strong inner relationship. One seminar participant had turtles who were becoming more and more lethargic. Eventually, it became very difficult to tell if the turtles were even alive. Someone knowledgeable with the Bach Flowers might have suggested Wild Rose or even Olive or Gorse. But the owner of the turtles intuitively gave her little loved ones Mustard, a flower with which she felt a strong inner relationship. The turtles came alive within twenty-four hours.

An abused dog recovers

Helena, our seven-year-old, mixed-breed female dog, shows distinct signs of a serious fear neurosis. We got her from a kennel, and she fears all people that she doesn't know, especially children. She doesn't accept any food from strangers and seems to be on her way to becoming a biter out of fear.

Prescription: Mimulus for fear of people and Star of Bethlehem for shock from the time spent in the kennel.

Report after a week: For the first time, Helena went to the neighbors' house, begging for food.

A blackbird is saved

One morning during the summer I woke up because of a strong blow against the terrace door. I found a blackbird lying on the terrace surrounded by some feathers. I could see traces of blood on the glass door where he had hit it hard. The bird's situation seemed hopeless. One had to pay close attention to even see his weak breathing. The position of his legs and claws was like that of a dead bird.

Since this was a situation that had to do with shock, I put a few drops of Rescue Remedy into a dish next to the bird, since I couldn't see a way to put any drops in his beak.

After about thirty minutes I checked on the bird and could see that he must have come into contact with the contents of the dish, since I could see a few drops on his feathers. I was hopeful. The blackbird was turning his head back and forth but not really moving from the spot. After another hour, more progress. Alert hops were peppered with short flights across the terrace. In the afternoon the "patient" succeeded in making longer flights, although the blackbird was always just within sight. It seemed like the bird was telling me: "I'm doing well, don't worry if you lose sight of me."

A cow gives milk again

During the birth of her calf, our cow must have had some sort of a shock, because she wouldn't give any milk. After about five days of Rescue Remedy drops, the cow started to give milk again, and even an extra liter a day.

Cat stories—Fina and Moppi

A lady who would pick up stray cats and try to find new homes for them helped many animals overcome illness and crises with the use of the Bach Flowers. Here are two experiences from her cat journal:

Fina came to me on July 7, 1974, as the first of my five cats (three females and two males, all with different parents). From the first moment we understood each other very well. She was very sensitive, but at the same time a loving and happy creature.

Since April of 1983 I knew she had liver problems and was also diabetic. The vet gave her medicine for the liver problem, but in the animal's interest I decided against treatment for diabetes. When Euli, another cat, died on June 16, 1983, Fina's state deteriorated markedly. In the next few weeks, it looked more and more as if she was nearing the end. I prepared a mixture of Walnut for the transition phase; Crab Apple for cleansing; and Rescue Remedy, Agrimony, and Centaury for her general diseased state. I gave her three drops three times daily. After a few doses she became quieter, but she would hardly take in solid food and would only drink. Smart little Fina, with whom I had spent so many wonderful times, left us on Sunday, June 27, 1983 without making a sound.

I once read that two little kittens come to pick up a cat's soul when it dies. That had to be so; Fina would always look toward the same direction, alternately snarling and hissing. Then she would look at me and purr. It seemed that she felt a threat getting closer and closer until she could no longer avoid it.

About two days before this happened I "saw" this cat, who had grown so close to my heart, as a small kitten playing around the hedge of a big house. She was jumping spiritedly around, and was happy and healthy. It seemed different than a dream, somehow more three-dimensional. The thought that there is care for animals even in another dimension was an inspiration and comfort for me.

Since December 1974 Moppi was the first tomcat in our cat community. He and Fina developed a friendship very quickly, which I think is not very common for cats. As far as I could tell, they were equals and were content with each other.

During this time we always had other animals who stayed as long as it took to find them a home. In retrospect, I think Moppi was always very happy when it was only him and his Fina, together. But, as time went by, there were three other animals that stayed with us constantly. Moppi turned into a little sheriff and constantly looked for a new spot to spray, a common tendency among cats. This is often an act of protest that pet owners misunderstand, and it often leads to animals losing their home. Luckily Moppi's "spray stations" were *mostly not in the house, otherwise I would have also had to face some unpleasant consequences.*

After Fina left us, I worried about Moppi. He didn't know what to do with himself, and would just sit for long periods of time and stare at the wall. His sadness also expressed itself in increased peeing. On September 21, 1983, I mixed a combination of Heather and Rescue Remedy drops. I gave him three drops twice a day. Soon I noticed a positive change. He conscientiously went to his litterbox and did not spray again. Now he is happy again, always wants to play with me, and makes his little jumps through the air.

Moving with plants

During my move, my plants didn't exactly get a very loving treatment by the moving company. Although I had specifically asked for extra care, and it had been promised to me, the plants were all wilting, many leaves had dropped, and some pots were even stacked on top of each other.

Before the move I had put Walnut on their stalks, in order to facilitate their transition. After the move I immediately added Rescue Remedy, Hornbeam, and Wild Rose to their water—Hornbeam and Rescue Remedy to aid against shock and for the strengthening of their stalks; Wild Rose because the plants had to submit without complaint to their fate. In the meantime, all the plants have recovered from the move, are blossoming again, and are feeling well in their new surroundings.

A leaf recovers

I brought an Aralie home from the market. One of its leaves was just hanging there, and even after two days there were no signs of improvement. I put Hornbeam, Olive, Walnut, and Wild Rose in the

watering can and watered the plant. I set the remaining water under
the withering leaf. Two hours later I glanced over at the plant and
was amazed; the leaf had recovered completely.

A fig tree in an involuntary winter sleep

*A small fig tree that I had outside during the summer had to be put
temporarily into the garage because there was an early frost, and I
hadn't prepared a place for it in the house yet. I had planned to bring
it into the house as soon as possible, but I inadvertently set it down in
a corner and unfortunately forgot about it.*

*Three months later I was cleaning the garage and came across
something I barely recognized as the little fig tree I had brought in. I
wasn't surprised to find it in such a state—without any leaves—since
it had been in low light, without much air, and kept at pretty much
around the freezing point all this time. I brought the plant into the
house to its designated place. Being an emergency situation, for sev-
eral days I gave it a few drops of Rescue Remedy with its water. That
was followed up with a treatment of Hornbeam for an entire week,
after which new shoots were apparent.*

*Four weeks of Bach Flower Therapy healed my little fig tree. Now
it's strong and healthy and covered with leaves and even some fruit.*

Parasites on the run

*A houseplant that I cared for very much began wilting unexplainably.
I put a Bach Flower mixture in its water: Rescue Remedy against environmental influences that might affect it; Wild Rose for its dying
leaves and flowers; and Crab Apple against possible vermin.*

*After three hours, I found a small maggot in the pot that had been
digging deviously around the root system. After three days of Bach
Flower treatment I found another small intruder, but the plant seems*

to be doing much better. The leaves don't hang lifelessly anymore, and there are a lot of full new blossoms. The small insects in the dirt don't seem to like the Bach Flower combinations very much. As a precaution, I will use Bach Flowers for a few more days, so that the plant can regain its strength completely.

A fir tree molts

I have two fir trees in my garden. When the trees began putting out new shoots, I noticed that one of the trees had yellowing needles and noticeably fewer shoots than the other one. It didn't look like it would make it through the summer.

As an experiment, I used Rescue Remedy for three days on the fir. Ten drops dissolved in a ten-liter bucket of water seemed to have an impressive effect after as little as four days. The tree recovered rapidly and in no time there was no difference between the two firs anymore.

5

EXPERIENCES
with Rescue Remedy

No other Bach Flower essence has generated so many reports of positive experiences as Rescue Remedy, the so-called First Aid drops. A mixture of Rock Rose, Star of Bethlehem, Clematis, Cherry Plum and Impatiens, Bach conceived of this remedy for the sole purpose of solving temporary states of inner stress, and not as a long term treatment. For short term use it has proven to be just what he envisioned, a popular restorative that shouldn't be absent from anybody's medicine cabinet.

Rescue Remedy as a preliminary therapy to subsequent individualized Bach Flower Therapies

A psychiatric clinic's head physician gives us the following report: *Although the First Aid drops are designed for short term relief only, there are situations when one has to prescribe a few days of regular dosage before one can even begin an individualized Bach Flower Therapy, because the patient, in his extreme psychic state, does not have the strength to deal with his weaknesses and conduct:*

A patient who came to us a few weeks ago had been admitted to a number of mental hospitals in the last five months, without any success. Her diagnosis was "psychotic episodes" that manifested themselves as powerful states of fear. Because of her two previous hospital stays— with which she associated a lot of disappointment and trauma—the patient was in a continuous nervous state.

The prescription was six drops of Rescue Remedy three times a day for five days. Concomitantly, the patient was also given homeopathic relaxants such as Avena, Sativa, and Chamomile.

After five days the patient was at least fifty percent more relaxed, which meant we could start an individualized Bach Flower Therapy that was very positive. This treatment continues today.

Rescue Remedy as a bridge to overcoming severe initial reactions in the beginning or during a Bach Flower Therapy

Following are notes from the diary of a patient in the first phases of therapy.

October 18: For the first time I fall asleep without any sleeping pills. Before I went to bed I had a glass of water with four drops of Rescue Remedy in it. I woke up without any fear. The morning goes well; I wash my hair and I feel good. Then uneasiness and states of panic begin again. I take Rescue Remedy. I feel pain in my chest again, but I rub some Rescue Remedy cream on it, which helps immediately.

Rescue Remedy as a rapid relaxant in daily medical and naturopathic practice

A naturopath from Hamburg writes:

Little Verena, four years old, comes to my office so I can draw some blood from her finger. It is not the first time she has been here; she knows the procedure and has always been very brave. Today it is different. Talking to her doesn't help—she screams very loud.

Then I remember the First Aid drops. I give her a small glass with a few drops in it. She takes a sip and then she takes a deep breath. I support this by saying, "Let's all take a deep breath." Verena starts to laugh and laugh, as if she wants to say "What's with all this commotion?" Now she lets me give her a small prick in her finger, the blood flows freely, and the procedure is over quickly.

Similar discoveries have been made by dentists, some of whom even give children and sensitive patients a glass with a few drops of Rescue Remedy as soon as they come to the office. The procedure progresses quite smoothly after that for both the patient and the dentist. The First Aid drops have proven successful for other practitioners as well. An Austrian massage therapist reports that she uses Rescue Remedy cream on her patients before and after each foot reflexology treatment, in order to cut down on the pain experienced at the more unpleasant points.

First Aid drops as a catalyst— to be used when a seemingly correct combination of Bach Flowers does not produce the expected effects

A man from Switzerland writes:
My father, who is eighty-five years old, has had a tendency toward depression all his life, but has always been able to help himself with his own philosophical way of looking at things. Only a few years ago, he said for the first time, "Today I am depressed." He refused any antidepressant that was offered to him. From February of 1982 on—since I've been reading Bach Flower Therapy—*I have been giving him Mustard. He did not feel any improvement. Then I tried Rescue Rem-*

edy which worked very well. He says his mood normalizes very quickly when he takes the Rescue Remedy drops.

Rescue Remedy—
even for periods when the energetic shock is already behind us

A naturopath from Northern Germany writes:

The patient, a thirty-eight-year-old doctor's aide started in September of 1981 to have strong pains in her groin area; her face was pale, and she suffered acute abdominal pains. She was taken to the hospital where she underwent surgery for a tubal pregnancy. Since this operation, from time to time she gets restless and fearful before her period. Her bleeding during her menstrual cycle has also been excessive.

In August of 1983, the patient came to my practice. Because her symptoms had all appeared since her operation, I deduced that we were dealing with a shock that hadn't been overcome yet, so I gave her Rescue Remedy drops.

After her next period, she told me that she had felt very well, and that even her family members were amazed by her balanced behavior. Menstrual bleeding is not so heavy for her any longer. Removal of her uterus—which had been planned—is no longer under consideration by either the patient or the doctor.

The First Aid drops as a foil for a critical situation during the course of a chronic illness

A Swiss woman writes:

My older sister has always had repeated fainting spells—after puberty, pregnancy, and menopause. It was only during menopause (about two years ago) that her situation finally received a medical diagnosis. She has had a heart valve defect since birth. The doctor suggested a difficult operation as a course of action, but my sister could not accept the risk and declined. As I became more familiar with Bach Flowers, I suggested Rescue Remedy as therapy at the first sign of a problem. She followed my advice with the result that she has been free of fainting spells for fourteen months now (except for one time when drops were not available). My sister is very happy. Her quality of life has improved with the removal of this burden.

Similar observations have been made by various people who care for the elderly, for example regarding states of restlessness experienced by sclerotic nursing home occupants.

Classic applications of Rescue Remedy

EXCITABLE STATES IN CHILDREN

My daughter Marie is twenty-two months old. She has a favorite shirt, with a certain label on it, that she always needs when she goes to sleep. She puts her thumb in her mouth and with the other hand she holds the shirt and strokes herself with the label.

One night we accidentally left the shirt at a friend's house. Marie started crying and I couldn't settle her down. I was getting ready to give her the Flower drops that she usually takes around this time when I noticed the Rescue Remedy next to her usual bottle. At the same time Marie pointed to the Rescue Remedy bottle and said, "I want that, Mommy." I thought that that was a good idea so I gave her some. A few moments later, Marie was relaxed and started looking at picture books with me. After about fifteen minutes she fell asleep, more relaxed than usual. She even took her thumb out of her mouth. Rescue Remedy should be present in every kindergarten.

BRUISES

As I was playing volleyball with my children, I jammed one of my fingers on my right hand against the ball. Naturally, it hurt a lot.

After an hour my finger was swollen and blue. That is when I remembered my Rescue Remedy cream and thought about all the cells that had gotten such a wicked shock. I put the salve on my finger.

I was flabbergasted the next day when the swelling and discoloration had disappeared. I could only feel a little pain. I used the cream again and, after two days, I couldn't feel anything anymore.

. .

I was renovating my house and as I bent over to pick up a piece of adhesive tape, I inadvertently banged my thumb into the wall. Immediately a bruise formed under my thumbnail and my thumb was in excruciating pain. I put Rescue Remedy cream on the bruise right away and the pain subsided very quickly. After half an hour I repeated the treatment, and a short time later I was able to hold something in my hand. The next day, even touching the nail was not that painful anymore.

. .

A very good, even astonishing, result occurred with the use of Rescue Remedy cream after catching my finger in a car door. Five minutes after application the pain was gone, and the next day the bruise also disappeared.

INSECT BITES
Last year in late fall I found a wasp on my desk. I put it outside through the window since, out of principle, I do not kill any animals. Two hours later, as I was putting on my coat jacket, I felt a powerful sting on my right arm, close to an artery. The wasp, whose life I had saved earlier, had returned in the arm of my blazer. It took some effort to get rid of her and to remove the stinger, so I could only apply the Rescue Remedy cream fifteen minutes later when I got home. I was

in pain for another hour or so, but there was never any swelling. The next day, I would have needed a magnifying glass to find the place where I had been stung.

BURNS
A naturopath writes:
I don't know if it was coincidence or divine providence that I read something about burns in Bach Flower Therapy *just before I had the following experience:*

Three weeks before Christmas a twelve-year-old boy suffered third-degree burns on his upper body. After emergency-room care and some treatment in the hospital, the conclusion was drawn that the only course of action would be skin grafts, sometime shortly before Christmas. In consulting with parents, it was obvious that they wanted to bypass the torture of skin grafts, but I was still skeptical about what I had read in the book about Rescue Remedy cream. Therefore we decided to let the hospital treatment continue, in conjunction with the cream, since I couldn't take the responsibility for a treatment exclusively with Rescue Remedy, not having had enough experience or information about the effect of the cream.

After about eight days there was a postponement of the skin graft operation. During this time, there had been an incredible granulation (new tissue growth around the wound) moving inward toward the burn center. During Christmas we didn't even consider the skin grafts anymore, and by the end of January the wound had closed completely. Unfortunately, neither I nor the parents had ever imagined the possibility of such a speedy recovery, so we don't have a pictorial record of the healing process.

STAGE FRIGHT
A professional consultant writes:
I find myself taking First Aid drops in situations that cause me anxiety—

such as radio shows, presentations, or speeches. The drops work wonders for me because I relax and so manage to make my point effectively.

MOTION SICKNESS
A report from a Swiss librarian:
For about two years I have been suffering from motion sickness, especially nausea and anxiety, when I fly, most often at takeoff and landing. During my last trip, as I was waiting for my flight, I took some Rescue Remedy, and on the plane before takeoff, some Scleranthus. Before landing I took them both together. I had no more symptoms.

As I was flying back from the Caspian Sea to Germany, our layover was uncertain due to some closed airports. Compared to the other passengers and to my earlier attitude, I was not as nervous or excited.

. .

On a flight from Zurich to Delhi, with a layover in Bombay, I was in the grip of terrible nausea. Various drugs did not help. After landing in Bombay, I was faced with the decision of whether I should continue with my flight to Delhi or ride out my indisposed state in a hotel. I reached for my Rescue Remedy drops. Within thirty minutes I had completely recovered.

Individual First Aid mixtures for special occasions

Practice has shown that individuals have characteristic "psychic emergency situations" caused by particular conditions. A typical character trait is as responsible as any external catalyst. In such cases, it would be worthwhile to prepare an individual First Aid mixture for a particular situation, in which one would add to Rescue Remedy the flower appropriate for the circumstances.

Examples:

- A divorced flight attendant works for the same airline as her ex-husband, who has a very strong personality. She has actually freed herself from him psychically, but the thought of having to interact with him professionally leaves her in states of anxiety similar to those she had at the end of their marriage.

    Personal First Aid mixture: Rescue Remedy, Honeysuckle (release from the past), and Walnut (guard against influence).

- A medical technician of retirement age feuds constantly with her landlady. Every disagreement quickly develops into an argument.

    Personal First Aid mixture: Rescue Remedy, Holly (inclination toward strong expressions of feelings), and Willow (she feels at the mercy of the landlady).

- The manager of a publishing company often wakes up around 3 A.M. in a panic-stricken state over difficult situations that will need to be faced that day.

    Personal First Aid mixture: Rescue Remedy and White Chestnut (thoughts he can't get rid off).

In acute states, the dosage of such mixtures can be increased to more than four drops. At the same time, as is always the case with Rescue Remedy, the dosage can be repeated after fifteen minutes if needed.

6

THE BACH FLOWERS
in the Medical and Natural Healing Practices

It is welcome news that, in spite of the overabundance of new forms of therapy being introduced all over the world, Bach Flower Therapy is being used not only by doctors and naturopaths but also by dentists and pharmacists, and is especially popular among younger age groups.

The unique therapeutical concepts for the treatment of character as set up by Dr. Edward Bach are recognized by many as something that they have been searching for a long time. Thoughts such as the following have been expressed quite often:

This therapy corresponds to my fundamental concept that every person has rights in illness, and that the person who treats the patient has no rights—in the sense of traditional medicine—to use unnecessary roughness in invading human development processes, or to do even more harm by not looking at the larger picture.

The Bach Flower Therapy reflects my interpretation of the therapist as a companion on the road to healing, an enabler between the physical illness and the soul. I would like to thank you for spreading the word about this therapy in the German-speaking countries; otherwise it probably would have been many years before it became known here.

Different interpretations of the role of therapist as adviser, or "travel companion on the train of Fate," become distinct in many letters. Most people who have shared their experiences with us have learned, as recommended, to accept the effect of the flowers as part of an extended process of therapy and self-discovery.

A Swiss naturopath writes:

Every person who intends to begin some form of Bach Flower Therapy should ask himself this question: "Why do I want to become healthy again, or just healthier than I am? So I can continue to be inconsiderate, angry, or jealous? Or should I learn from my suffering to be a better person toward myself and my fellow man?" You cannot do justice to your recovery if you haven't earned your health!

A different colleague writes:

I believe an individual's inner state has an important influence on the kind of emotional energy frequency with which the Bach Flower combinations will become associated. In the final analysis, whether a therapy is successful or not depends on the will of the patient. That is why I always recommend that my patients do something to support the therapy structure. In this way they help themselves, even if only symbolically, to support the healing process.

Naturally, because of the many demands we face on a daily basis, it is hard to allow ourselves to become as fully immersed in the

Flower Therapy as desired. When this frustration occurs, consulting the questionnaire in the appendix may be of help. Patients may take it home, or even fill it out in the waiting room. By conscientiously analyzing questionnaire results, the patient should be able to choose the correct Bach Flower Remedies with at least 90 percent accuracy. In any case, this is much more reliable and, in the spirit of "heal thyself," a lot more meaningful for the patient compared to a battery of comprehensive tests and measurements in which the patient typically assumes a passive role.

If one does not experience any breakthroughs on the first try with a Flower Therapy, one must not become discouraged. There must be a reason that prevents us from recognizing the necessary flower.

A doctor from Southern Germany writes:

> I am under the impression, from personal experience, that very often there is one particular flower that will set recovery in motion. Without this one, the other flowers will have a limited effect, even if they were chosen correctly.

At this point it is important to reiterate that the Bach Flower Remedies may be combined with all other forms of therapy, even with the high-power treatments of classic homeopathic medicine. Very good results were obtained in combining Bach Flowers with low- to medium-potency homeopathic remedies, Schussler salts, snake enzymes, or anthroposophic remedies. However, for purely technical, observational reasons, it is not recommended that anyone follow a Bach Flower Therapy concurrently with a high-potency homeopathic treatment.

Classic homeopaths have often come into contact with Bach Flowers and have insisted that this therapy depends upon the determination of a singular, optimal flower essence. This, however, does not correspond to the school of thought that each individual situation is best treated by a unique constellation of energy influences on psychic states.

The majority of doctors or naturopaths who use Bach Flowers in their practices do so in combination with other forms of therapy; the Flowers have proven positive in these instances. Following are four quotations typifying the success of the Bach Flower Remedies when used in conjunction with other forms of treatment.

> I use the Flowers as an addition to classic homeopathic remedies, and I have a lot of success with them. The search for the appropriate Bach Flower allows other factors to surface, which aids in finding an appropriate homeopathic remedy as well.

. .

> My experiences with Bach Flowers have been remarkable, and I am of the opinion that before any therapy one should also take a Bach Remedy. When the spiritual and psychic suppression of negative states is set in motion, it makes half of all other drugs superfluous. Furthermore, I have noticed that the presence of a Bach Flower will speed up the effect of other drugs.

. .

> I have noticed that the Bach Flowers open passage to a "healing road," which shortens the time that one has to take drugs.

. .

> Time and again I have noticed—and I strongly believe—that with the use of the Bach Flowers there is a tendency for the state of the patient to become harmonized more quickly, and therefore subsequently prescribed methods of treatment have a better effect.

The following case studies of acute and chronic states have been documented by doctors and naturopaths. In each situation, Bach

Flowers have been used either exclusively or in conjunction with other forms of therapy.

Bach Flowers for the
natural inducing of labor

The patient, Elke S., is a twenty-four-year-old graphic artist. Elke took Bach Flowers throughout her problem-free pregnancy. Her motivation was her wish for further development of her character and support for the prenatal development of her child. For the delivery, she looked for a hospital where she could have a natural birth.

At the end of her eighth month, her water broke unexpectedly one night. In the morning she went to the hospital where, by late afternoon, with no apparent labor pains, the decision was made to induce labor by the next day at the latest. Since this was contradictory to her desire to experience natural childbirth, she called me wanting to know if Bach Flowers would be a good idea under these circumstances. I considered the following:

Since the mother had been using Bach Flowers throughout her entire pregnancy and felt relaxed and in a good frame of mind, we had to concentrate more on the condition of the child, who apparently wasn't ready to wrestle his way into existence.

What kind of feelings could the baby be experiencing? Fear of the world (Mimulus). Vacillating between two possibilities (Scleranthus). Indecision of ambitions (Wild Oat). Absence of energy, for the taking of a decisive last step (Walnut).

A mixture of these four flowers was prescribed with a dosage of three drops hourly for five hours. After her third dose at nine o'clock in the evening, light labor pains set in. By midnight she was in active labor. Fifty minutes later her son was born. He is an extremely vital child—a characteristic I have observed in most "Flower babies."

Fear of enrollment in school

A six-year-old boy was afraid of enrolling in school. His fear only in-creased as the enrollment day grew nearer. His mother took him to the pediatrician, who prescribed a sedative, but, according to his mother, his fearful, whining state did not change. Particularly in the evening, before going to bed, the child's fears manifested themselves in the form of crying, feelings of discouragement, and the words "I am not going to school."

I chose the following flowers: Mimulus, for fear of known things; Aspen, for vague fears; and Elm, for the feeling of not being up to the task.

The boy's therapy began one week before school was supposed to start. As early as two days later, a change had occurred in him. He was calmer, more relaxed, and showed interest in school. On the first day of school, as his mother tells it, he went to school full of joy and everything was fine.

After the first bottle was used up, I examined the recipe again and re-placed Elm with Clematis so the boy could pay better attention in school. When I checked with his parents again, I was told that their son had adapted well to school and there were no more occasions of restlessness.

A student overcomes her instability
and a dependence on hashish

An eighteen-year-old student grew up with her younger sister and their mother—who was pretty young herself—under a certain amount of deprivation, in an apartment in a large city. The father had left their mother when the patient was still very young.

She had feelings of hate for her mother, was inactive, and just bummed around. She was dependent on hashish. Her mother said she had an almost obsessive need for cleanliness, and she would never touch a foreign towel.

On February 7, I prescribed the following Flower combination: Star of Bethlehem, for overcoming the shock of the separation from her father and the earlier violent disagreements between her parents;

Holly, for the feelings of hate toward her mother and society in general; Hornbeam, for lack of internal incentive and the misconception that she can only function if she smokes; and Crab Apple, for her obsessive cleanliness urges.

On March 1st, she was doing a little better. By April 11, she was a lot more active and participated in sports. She didn't seem to smoke hashish anymore and even avoided the company of the "no future" crowd. On May 31, I prescribed the same combination again, in order to stabilize the positive states. At the end of June, her mother called me and reported, "I am very happy with my daughter. She has found a new joy in life."

Neurovegetative disturbances in anticipation of divorce proceedings

A fifty-one-year-old massage therapist came to me in May of 1983 with complaints of nervous heart palpitations, headaches associated with her period, problems with her veins, and stool irregularity.

Patient's history: She had married late and had her first son at the age of forty-one. Her present problems were due to a loss of strength because of earlier liver, gall, and kidney diseases. Initially she had been a very vital individual, but because of her illnesses she could no longer care for her husband—he being the "needy child" type—and he started looking at other women and had filed for divorce three years earlier. On top of her physical condition, this was something that the patient could only marginally deal with.

Before the start of the Bach Flower Therapy, the patient was treated with traditional allopathic medicines to help with menstruation problems, for the support of the kidney, which had shown to be sensitive in the reflex areas, and for nervous heart conditions. During the entire course of the therapy, we also introduced discussion sessions and foot reflexology.

During our sessions, the patient chose the following Bach Flowers:

- *Vine was in this case not typical of her character and situation, but it was needed as support, because the patient had the strong will to overcome her current emotional and financial problems. She tried to compensate for her frailty by dealing with the outside world with excessive hardness and severity.*
- *Star of Bethlehem had a very positive effect on her nervous heart condition, as well as her menstrual discomfort, so that I could discontinue the allopathic medicines as permanent remedies, and only use them occasionally.*
- *Cherry Plum—The patient had been a bed wetter as a child, and in this parting situation she was afraid of letting go emotionally. She suffered often from various cramps and spasms that subsided, however, during the course of the treatment.*
- *Willow—During her marriage, the patient had given up everything that had initially given her pleasure. Willow would also alleviate her menstrual problems.*
- *Gentian—The patient was skeptical, easily discouraged, and disappointed.*
- *Crab Apple—The patient was disgusted by pimples and sweat; she couldn't relax and her solar plexus was often tightened up.*

After about four weeks of therapy, the patient got short-term cramps in the gall area which she treated herself by massage and reflexology, making them disappear in about two hours. She reiterated during her last visit that she had never felt as well as in the last few weeks, and had not remembered that anyone could feel so light and relieved. She had even rejoined her old church group for choir practice.

By November of 1983, the patient seldom experienced any kind of heart discomfort and her menstrual problems had been cured. Her relationship with her son, which had been very difficult after the separation, was improving. She had resigned herself to the upcoming divorce.

Drug withdrawal therapy with support from Bach Flower Remedies

The patient, male, late thirties, has been using drugs for eight years: hashish for the first five years, and later heroin. After that he abused various prescription drugs such as codeine and Valium.

Patient's history: He was adopted, parents unknown, and during childhood was exposed to an abusive adoptive father. He took a job as a cabin boy, set out to sea, but eventually became unemployed, studied to become a salesman but didn't like it. He stepped out of the mainstream, hung out with a gang, and started taking drugs. There was an attempt at rehabilitation, but the withdrawal symptoms were too powerful, and therapy was interrupted.

Before the rehabilitative withdrawal therapy began, the patient had been pretreated with Bach Flowers for nine months, in order for him to be stabilized and emotionally motivated to work through the rehabilitation process and all the withdrawal symptoms that come with it. Unfortunately, the exact prescriptions used during this phase were not documented.

There were mixtures of "fear" flowers, such as Aspen, Cherry Plum, and Rock Rose, because the patient was in constant fear of not getting enough pills. Because those thoughts were hounding him I added White Chestnut. For his weak emotional state I gave him Wild Rose, Gorse, Sweet Chestnut, Star of Bethlehem. And finally, Larch as well, because he feared he couldn't finish his rehabilitation.

Main phase of treatment: the actual withdrawal therapy started on January 10: no more drugs, no more alcohol. For the physical aspect of treatment, high Vitamin B-complex dosage, Hypericum D2 and Quarz D6, Nux Vonica C200, Avena Sativa tincture, Cardums

Marianus tincture, and Bach Flower drops were introduced.
   The Bach Flower combinations:

- *Agrimony—as a catalyst for the ability to confront the unpleasant, hovering, dark side of ourselves and of life*
- *Clematis—release from the make-believe world, the twilight of intoxication, in order to have one's feet on solid ground again*
- *Gentian—because the Flower Therapy patient still has doubts*
- *Crab Apple—for the feeling of physical and emotional uncleanliness and for the excretion of such poisons*
- *Olive—since the patient has reached a limit to his emotional and physical energies, and in the absence of deafening impulses has to soberly recognize his painful state of being*
- *Walnut—(in connection with Gentian)—as a catalyst for a possible breakthrough to a life without drugs, for a radical new reorientation*

Course of therapy: The beginning was characterized by very strong emotional and physical pain, but the goodwill of the patient, activated by the Flower Therapy, opened him up to intensive meditation sessions, in which he tackled some emotional reconditioning of his past.

By January 17, 1984, the patient no longer suffered from withdrawal symptoms. I set up a new prescription for flower combinations: Honeysuckle, Pine, Star of Bethlehem, White Chestnut, Cherry Plum, and Agrimony.

New stages of development were in full swing. The patient was intensively reexamining his past (Honeysuckle) and couldn't comprehend how he managed to spend eight years of his life involved with drugs.

This phase resulted in strong feelings of self-blame (Pine). Many shocking experiences from his past, including childhood, now became quite conscious (Star of Bethlehem). An overwhelming insomnia pointed to the fact that he was overwrought with thoughts and images

(White Chestnut). This sudden overload of images had to be controlled so it wouldn't give rise to new fears and aggressions (Cherry Plum). Confrontation with the self and with the laws of everyday life has to be supported in order to prevent eventual tendencies for a renewed spiritual flight or escape (Agrimony).

Today the patient is well, looks much younger, and is making plans for the future. His therapy continues.

Difficulties in the area of social interaction, accompanied by asthmatic complaints and rashes

This case study comes from a combined doctor and psychologist practice.

Thirty-six-year-old Armgard came to us because she had difficulty making contact with other people. In addition, this masculine-appearing woman was suffering from itchy rashes which, as soon as they subsided, would make way for asthmatic problems.

Patient's history: Armgard was unmarried and lived in the same orphanage in which she sought shelter with her grandmother when she was eight years old and fled the former East Germany. She was the cook for the orphanage, where she apprenticed as a young girl in the kitchen, but she had no formal education.

Armgard saw at least four or five doctors at the same time: internists, dermatologists, gynecologists, and others. A naturopath dealt with her complaints about disks, and a gynecologist with her abdominal problems and headaches.

We included her in one of our therapeutic discussion groups, hoping she would learn to overcome her difficulties in interacting with others. At the same time we treated her with Bach Flowers.

Armgard's main problem at work was that she was very surly to children and coworkers, and therefore nobody cared for her very much. She would lose her temper very quickly and naturally experienced problems because of it. She sang in the church choir, played the flute, and took pottery classes, but never made contact with the people that she met there. She fought her sleeping problems with beer and whiskey.

Course of therapy: During our discussion groups, it was a year before Armgard came out of herself, took any stand in conversation, or even engaged someone else in conversation. In the course of her two-year treatment with the Bach Flowers, she used four different mixtures. Selections were based on conversations or chosen spontaneously (grabbing) by the patient.

In the first phase we prescribed, in response to her negative emotional state, Cherry Plum, Sweet Chestnut, and Impatiens. Since she tended to manifest this state outwardly we added Agrimony. For her physical and emotional exhaustion, which she tried to compensate with an overbearing will, she also got Olive and Vervain.

During the second phase the patient showed progress in dealing with emotional problems. Olive and Agrimony were kept in the recipe. For her current feelings of fear and inferiority we included Mimulus, Larch, and White Chestnut. Wild Oat was added because Armgard began thinking about her work and mission in life. The inner process was quickly becoming more intense.

In the third phase we used Honeysuckle (for breaking away from her past), Sweet Chestnut (she was obviously at a crossroads), Walnut (the need for change), and Aspen and Crab Apple (for the avoidance of influences that needed to be left behind). The last two flowers were also included in an effort to alleviate asthmatic complaints and skin problems. This third combination brought about the decisive breakthrough that would be stabilized in the fourth phase.

Fourth phase: We continued with Honeysuckle, Walnut, and Crab Apple. We added Chestnut Bud (so she didn't fall back on behavioral patterns that hinder progress), and Red Chestnut (for the final dissolution of the image of her grandmother as her strongest point of reference).

Status after two years: Armgard's skin problems have not recurred.

Her headaches are gone. In her work environment she is happy and accepted by others. She is also interested in gymnastics, pays attention to her wardrobe, and admits to being more in command of her personal affairs. Her only problems are occasional breathing difficulties. Her numerous visits to the doctor have also stopped. We cannot say for a fact which flower caused a particular result, but the fact is that Armgard is now doing better than at any time in her life.

Back pain with chronic feelings of fear and exhaustion

A forty-three-year-old butcher came to my office on October 4, 1983, because of back pain associated with strong feelings of fear.

Patient's history: When the patient was a child, his father shot his mother and then committed suicide. He grew up in various foster homes, partly with relatives, partly with strangers. He never felt loved and started working at an early age in a butcher shop.

Symptoms and prescribed Bach Flowers: Unexplained fear of impending doom. Sometimes while driving his throat would closed up (Aspen). At work he easily became irritated with his apprentices and employees (Impatiens). Fourteen- to sixteen-hour workdays exhausted him, but he kept on working (Oak). He could not get over the violent deaths of his parents (Star of Bethlehem).

After about six weeks the patient seemed to be in a better state, more balanced. This has continued, even after terminating the Bach Flower drops, until today (February, 1984). For his back trouble, the patient is currently in specialized therapy.

Sleep disturbances with nightly urges for movement

The patient, Dieter K., a fifty-five-year-old sales manager, had been diabetic for quite a while. He didn't have any illnesses, but for two years he had complained about depression and peculiar sleeping patterns. He fell asleep easily, but woke up exactly one hour later with strong feelings of fear that only subsided if he got up, went outside, and walked around the block. Then would go back to bed and fall asleep promptly. After an hour the episode would repeat itself. This happened up to six times per night. He was understandably nervous and, although very athletic and strong, his nerves were shot. This also started to affect his business dealings. Later he developed a strong inferiority complex.

The patient had tried everything possible in his visits to allopathic doctors and naturopaths, even acupuncture and laser therapy, all unsuccessfully.

Even I don't make any headway with the usual homeopathic, or even anthroposophic, treatments until I start Bach Flower Therapy. Rock Rose was as decisive as ever. Introduced as the only mode of treatment, it removed some of the anxiety from the states of fear. I continued with Mimulus, which at first exacerbated the sleeping problems. Some anxiety was still there at night, but at least it didn't involve getting out of bed anymore. I alternated Aspen and Agrimony with Mimulus and Rock Rose. After a long conversation I added Star of Bethlehem, and later White Chestnut.

After half a year, the patient was free of symptoms. The therapy continued, but with greater periods of time between consultations.

Impaired speech resulting from shock and anger

A seventy-nine-year-old retiree got involved in a spirited political discussion the day before elections. This resulted in a state of anxiety and during his disagreement with the younger crowd he felt himself grow quite fatigued. From that day on he began to lose his speech. Eight weeks later he came to my office because of continuing speech difficul-

ties. He said, "I have trouble saying anything. On top of that I feel very weak and listless and I've lost my appetite."

I prescribed Star of Bethlehem because of the emotional trauma that he had suffered. Eight days later he could speak better and his appetite had returned. The lump in his throat disappeared. He solved crossword puzzles again and had a renewed will to live. Ten days later, his speech problems had completely disappeared.

A geriatric case

An eighty-two-year-old recipient of social assistance had been complaining for weeks about pains in her abdominal area. The patient had been living for about ten years with her daughter, and they did not get along; there was a lot of arguing and the mother was jealous of her daughter's friends. She complained a lot, was very fearful, and had dreams about dying. Because of her stomach complaints she had spent three weeks in a hospital for tests. The results were inconclusive, and she was discharged. She became despondent and whiny and talked about death. The following flower combinations were prescribed:

- *Rock Rose—for her fears and nightmares*
- *Crab Apple—for the cramping of her solar plexus and her obsession with minor details*
- *Impatiens—for restlessness, impatience, and losing her temper quickly*
- *Heather—because she craved attention and exaggerated her state*
- *Holly—for her envy, jealousy, and dissatisfaction; she always saw the worst in things and always acted hurt*

Course of therapy: On the second day of Flower Therapy the patient's pains disappeared completely, even though she did not particularly believe in the flowers. She became more patient, relaxed, and from then on was easy to take care of.

Final stages of terminal illness

A forty-one-year-old man, with inoperable intestinal cancer, was released from the hospital at the request of his relatives, since he wished to die at home. His doctor had been treating him with homeopathic medicine, but his psychic condition was understandably pitiful. I prescribed a combination of flowers to give back his inner peace:

- *Gorse—for despair*
- *Cherry Plum—for the fear of letting go*
- *Holly—principle of love*
- *Rock Rose—for panic attacks*
- *Star of Bethlehem—for shocks and disappointments*

I prescribed four drops six times daily. After using up a thirty-milliliter bottle, I adjusted the combination by replacing Rock Rose and Star of Bethlehem with Walnut (breaking through to a new phase).

The patient's disposition changed markedly. He became more balanced, open, and thankful. Eight weeks after his return from the hospital he died fully alert, a word of thanks on his lips. His relatives were firm believers that the peace this dying man exuded was a result of the Flower Therapy.

A severely disabled
young man and his mother

This case was treated by both a doctor and a psychologist.
Bert, twenty-four years old, had been cared for at home by his mother since birth. During the day he was looked after in a therapy center.

Diagnosis: severe disability and retardation. The patient used a wheel-chair and had limited use of his hands. He had been subjected to an EEG (electroencephalogram) three times, having panic attacks each time. On the basis of the EEG, the doctors concluded the patient wasn't even viable. Presumably, his panic attacks influenced the data in a negative way. Bert is the third of four children and was born prematurely due to a fall by his mother. Before the beginning of Bach Flower Therapy, he had been treated with Convulex and Neuleptil, which had not brought about any ameliora-tion of his state. Both drugs were continued in reduced doses after the start of the Flower Therapy.

Symptoms: Bert woke up five or six times a night and had to have his position changed. During the day he was very aggressive, and would physically attack his mother, mostly by biting her. He flew into rages when he didn't get what he wanted. Bach Flower Therapy was started at his mother's request, for her son as well as for herself, since she had had very good experiences with the Rescue drops in extreme situations. The diagnosis was established based on discussions with the mother and through psychological observations.

First prescription for the mother:

- *Olive—for physical and emotional exhaustion*
- *Pine—for feelings of guilt, of not being able to do better*
- *Gorse—for deeply smoldering despair*
- *Star of Bethlehem—for the great shock suffered after delivery in finding out that her son would not be healthy*
- *Elm—for the feeling of not being able to cope with the responsibility*

First prescription for the son:

- *Rock Rose—for periods of panic. Since being accidently dropped once (Star of Bethlehem) he was afraid of every movement (Mimulus).*

- *Holly—for jealous tendencies and strong aggression, such as biting*
- *Heather—for general physical and emotional needs*
- *Rescue—every night for restlessness*

Observations after four weeks: the state of both patients had improved visibly. Bert slept through the night more often, and his mother felt like a weight had been lifted off her shoulders. On the basis of this relaxed situation the parents decided, for the first time in many years, to take a vacation and leave Bert with a caregiver.

Second prescription for the mother:

- *Continued with Olive and Elm. In addition, Larch—to stabilize her consciousness*
- *Red Chestnut—for the fear and worries about her son's future: "What will happen to him?"*
- *Gentian—for skepticism and tending toward hopelessness*

Second prescription for the son:

- *Continued with Star of Bethlehem, Rock Rose, Holly, and Heather*
- *In addition: Willow—for feelings of bitterness, of being in a hopeless situation*
- *Later: Impatiens—for inner impatience, restlessness, and excitable states*

Situation after six months: Bert continued to make progress. He slept even better, woke up around 4 A.M., and fell asleep again, needing only to be moved once or not at all. In the morning, his mother only had to look after him a couple of times. His aggression was sharply reduced; he bit very rarely. Most importantly, Bert was now approachable and seemed to understand when he couldn't have his way.

The patient's mother experienced a strengthening of her own emotional and physical states. Her outlook on life became more open and positive. She believed that the Bach Flower Therapy she and her son had been undergoing had had a positive effect on their lives. She was more relaxed and confident. More importantly, she accepted the situation and the role she played within it.

The Bach Flowers as support for the therapy of a POS child

A special education teacher from Switzerland reported:

Markus, who was ten years old, had been in my classroom for three years. He was a POS child (Psycho-Organic Syndrome, an infantile delay of brain development) who got discouraged very easily and was very fearful. Markus had trouble controlling his emotions and would subject everybody to violent outbursts. The smallest experience which he perceived as negative would disturb his emotional balance. He had trouble dealing with mishaps and had very low self-confidence. With a heavy heart, I had to refer him to one of my colleagues in April of 1983. In order to facilitate his transition, I suggested the Bach Flower Therapy to his mother, with which I had had such success in the past. Together with his mother and the naturopath who was going to treat him, we set up the following combination:

- *Chestnut Bud—for slow learning*
- *Gentian—for being easily discouraged*
- *Mimulus—for known fears*

Markus responded well to this combination, and so we continued it along with other flowers. Markus mostly chose the flowers himself through intuitive grabbing. In addition he got a so-called "school mix-

ture" consisting of Larch, Mimulus, and White Chestnut, which he felt was very supportive.

Beginning in March of 1984, Markus became very alert and kept up with school despite his learning disability. He became more responsible and independent. His earlier outbursts (yelling, aggression against classmates, despair, etc.) became very rare. He was not fearful of everything new anymore, and instead he had a lot more confidence.

For his parents, this transformation was a miracle, one that resulted in a more relaxed atmosphere in the home. For me, Markus's case represented a classic example of the success one can achieve with Bach Flower Therapy.

Bach Flower Therapy in a case of early-childhood autism and epilepsy

The patient, Peter, came from a family of pharmacists and was twenty-five years old.

Patient's history: normal birth with nothing noticeable happening in his first years until he developed a gradual delay in his speech development and a partial inability to play.

When Peter was five a child psychiatrist diagnosed early-childhood autism. At age eight, Peter was enrolled in a special school for the learning disabled. There, Peter had difficulty picking up basic school lessons. At eleven, he was in a day school for the mentally impaired. When he was sixteen he joined a workshop for disabled people. It was here that his first epileptic seizure occurred. His seizures recurred but with no particular pattern. In his seventeenth year he often experienced headaches and had aggressive behavior and depression. Peter would hit himself and others, destroy objects around him, and rip books apart. He could no longer stay at the workshop. His parents decided to care for him at home.

During this entire time no allopathic drugs were used, only

natural remedies like Baldrian, Melisse, various Strath preparations, but most of all PK7 (a yeast preparation) and vitamins, especially B-complex.

When Peter was nineteen the family moved to Schleswig-Holstein from Niedersachsen. Peter remained in home care. From 1979 to 1982, a special therapy which employs the use of electric frequencies (impulses and oscillations) for lymph cleansing and subtle mood changes was introduced. Peter's reactions varied from more aggressive to very harmonious.

On April 1, 1982, Bach Flower Therapy was started. The electric frequencies treatment had to be stopped, however, since—according to the therapist—his highly deranged nervous system was being too stimulated and therefore the subtle effects of the flower frequencies could not be appraised correctly.

Course of therapy: The treatment lasted for a period of about two years, during which time the use of many Bach Flowers was employed. Since intuitive grabbing was not possible due to the patient's condition, the prescriptions were established primarily through discussions with Peter's mother.

In 1982, the following key Flowers were typical in a prescription:

- Star of Bethlehem—because the faulty development was probably triggered by a series of emotional shocks at an extremely sensitive young age
- Sweet Chestnut—for inner despair
- Scleranthus—for strong inner hesitations
- Rock Rose—for very high nervous irritability
- Pine—for feelings of guilt
- Vine—for the desire to be able to prove himself

Besides the natural remedies given to him by his parents during his therapy, Peter was also treated with various Schussler salts, such as Aconitum.

Reactions: At first Peter started sleeping a lot; occasionally there would be tremendous pressure on his bladder, and he couldn't hold it in. His epileptic seizures were becoming more severe, with wetting also present. On the other hand, his almost daily headaches began subsiding.

In 1983 an entirely new group of flowers was prescribed in addition to those from the previous year. These new flowers were important because they pointed toward an awakening of Peter's own personality:

- *Honeysuckle*—for separation from the past
- *Red Chestnut*—for dissolution of a constricting band
- *Aspen*—for stabilizing of vague fears brought about by atmospheric influences
- *Holly*—for working through feelings
- *Walnut*—for breakthrough to a new developmental state

Reactions: Peter still slept a lot. This was interpreted as a sign that hard work was being done on an emotional plane. Wetting still occured during seizures, however, these episodes came about less often, were not as powerful, and passed quickly. Recovery time after a seizure was hardly needed anymore. Worthy of note is the fact that Peter's demeanor before the seizures, in comparison to earlier days, was marked by striking harmony.

His fears and aggression also became milder. He did not hit, hardly ever destroyed anything, and his coercive demeanor became more flexible. The pressure on his bladder manifested itself periodically, but his headaches disappeared. During 1983 Peter's psychic behavior varied, at times introverted and at other times harmonious and lively. His inner struggles were apparent. "I don't want to" was a common phrase. At other times he was willing to do everything required of him—a trip to the bathroom, a walk outside, etc. Depression

*set in occasionally, but dissolved after he had a good cry. One got the
impression that Peter's personality was developing within established
confines. To outsiders Peter seemed somehow childish and spiritless until 1983, and then suddenly he became more mature. A delicate mus-
tache appeared. When the therapist asked "How old are you?" he answers spontaneously, "Seventeen years old." That corresponded to his
outed habitus (he was actually twenty-five years old). The fact that
healing on an emotional plane had begun is shown in the following
observation: Peter always used to listen to very loud rock music. After
treatment he prefers more harmonious sounds, such as classical music,
opera, and choral music. His mother wrote: "Since the beginning of
Bach Flower Therapy, a lot of things have started to happen for
Peter, and I bless the day that we were able to start this therapy."*

After a seven-year interruption, a twenty-three-year-old menstruates again

*A somewhat withdrawn twenty-three-year-old legal aide, still living
at home with her parents, had had a normal menstrual cycle from
the age of twelve, when it first started, until the age of fifteen. After
an uneventful three-week trip to England that year her period became
irregular. When she was sixteen, it stopped altogether. Hormone treatments were ineffective and were stopped. Also unsuccessful were remedies such as Feminon and Agnolyt.*

*I prescribed four flowers that had more than average success in
such cases to be taken for eight weeks:*

- *Star of Bethlehem—for state of shock on a subtle energy plane*
- *Pine—for self-blame*
- *Rock Water—for rigid inner principles that suppress vital needs*
- *Cherry Plum—for fear of letting go inside*

In addition, the following flowers were prescribed for seven weeks:

- *Centaury—for lack of development of one's own will*
- *Walnut—the flower that succeeds with breakthrough*

The following is a description of the entire therapy in the patient's own words. It is a typical example of a classic course of a Bach Flower Therapy.

1st day, December 2, Friday:

Nothing out of the ordinary, some elation over the last couple of days (my trip to Hamburg, new acquaintances). I feel somewhat freer than usual.

2nd day, Saturday:

After waking up, I remember a dream I had in which I noticed that there was blood on my slip. I asked myself, incredulously, if it could be my period. I remember coming to the conclusion in the dream that it had to be my period. At this point I woke up, unable to see how my sensational discovery affected me in my dream. During the day, I feel a little more self-conscious than most days, state my opinion more often, and am no longer fearful about other people's reactions.

3rd day, Sunday:

More confident mood, otherwise unchanged.

4th day, Monday:

Feeling a little off, am leaning toward depression and a bad mood and am a little listless. I don't give in to my negative moods and eventually I overcome them.

8th day, Friday:

A part of me has a great trust in God and a wonderful feeling of happiness, and I feel His presence. Unfortunately, I felt discouraged and frightened earlier, but managed to suppress the feelings of guilt that this caused.

9th and 10th days, Saturday and Sunday:

I pay too much attention to other peoples' needs. My own then come up short. When I focus on my own sensibilities I get a bad conscience, feeling that I will hurt other people. Besides, my beliefs are quite firmly set.

11th day, Monday:

I have a new perspective at work. I am sure that my path is being shown to me, and I am being led down it even if it has some detours.

In the last three days I have had dreams that are more intense and lively. There are instances when I feel God's power in me, and I am calm and relaxed.

12th day, Tuesday:

Something has gone wrong. This time I cannot get out of, and lose myself in, my depression. God, lead me.

13th day, Wednesday:

I am discouraged and listless.

14th day, Thursday:

My depressive mood has increased. I feel indifferent and discouraged. My life seems bland and with no hope of improvement. I hope this is just an initial reaction to the Bach Flowers; I can take it.

15th day, Friday:

I have the feeling that life is empty; there is no hope and everything stagnates. I am not content with myself and have feelings of guilt.

It is worse than yesterday, but I continue to hope.

16th day, Saturday:

Just like yesterday, nothing seems to make any sense; however, I have this feeling deep inside that everything will change, but it's not very strong.

17th day, Sunday:

My mood is improving. I know I have to have patience. I am inspired to start taking piano lessons again and to study Italian. I know that the true lesson that I need to learn will be shown to me when the time is right, which it is not yet. I am aware now of times when I seem to slip into my old habit of only paying attention to the needs of others. That for me is a step forward. Unfortunately, I cannot seem to repress the feeling of guilt that I get every time my own desires are satisfied.

18th day, Monday:

It is a black day, empty, with depressive impulses.

19th day, Tuesday:

My mood has improved somewhat. I have renewed hope, but I continue to be disinterested and apathetic.

20th day, Wednesday:

Mood similar to yesterday, and I can feel that positive powers are working for me and guiding me. I become impatient and have to fight this feeling. I continue to hope, though. I know I will get what is coming to me.

21st day, Thursday:

I know where it's at, and I also know that my path is getting harder, but happier and more fulfilling.

22nd day, Friday:

My elevated mood has deflated somewhat, but I am confident and sure of myself.

23rd day, Saturday, Christmas Eve:

Nothing much has changed. I feel like I can't see very well, but I feel freer than before and am very confident.

24th day, Christmas Day:

I feel great strength and I hope I can use it sensibly.

At home I feel constrained, locked up. I want to force my fears and weaknesses. I want to move out and live my own life.

25th day, Monday:

Good mood overall, but with the feeling that everything is stagnant. I become impatient again.

26th day, Tuesday:

More and more I feel that I have to leave home. I feel locked up.

27th day, Wednesday:

I see better now. Otherwise, I am at a low point again; not an actual depression, but my old indolence returns.

28th day, Thursday:

No change.

29th day, Friday:

Partly in a good mood, but at home I feel cramped.

30th day, Saturday:

I am upset because I'm afraid of getting into a situation where I am unprotected, but I don't let myself fall under the influences of others.

31st day, January 1, 1984:

Definite stagnation. Something has to change, but I don't move one step forward. Even though I am afraid of being alone, I have to move out of the house.

32nd day, Monday:

Situation remains fairly unchanged. I demand change, progress, and development, but according to the outer circumstances everything is the same. Deep inside me, though, I feel that soon something will change. It's as if something which is simmering very quietly deep inside will come out powerfully sooner or later.

33rd day, Tuesday:

I am irritable, revert to old behavioral patterns, and get upset over it.

34th day, Wednesday:

I have a pretty good disposition today. I don't really know what to say here, but throughout the day I had certain premonitions that came true. No earth-shattering occurrences, but still I was quite amazed.

35th day, Thursday:

I woke up because of a peculiar dream. I don't know much more about it, but this is the scene imprinted on my memory:

I am in a traffic circle and I am searching for the correct street that will take me to my goal (I don't know exactly what it is, but I think I am looking for somebody important). Just as I decide on a certain street that I feel is the correct one, I sense a higher power leading me toward a different street, which turns out to be the right one. I am amazed, but at the same time not, since I feel it is God's guidance.

This dream is so clear in my mind. I interpreted it as being God—against my wisdom—showing me, or about to show me, the right way.

All this despite my inner doubts and resistance because of my fears. Otherwise, I am freer in dealing with other people. I still find it difficult to express my opinions clearly, but I have more tolerance toward myself and my mistakes.

36th day, Friday:

A little depressed, but not a lot. Actually, full of confidence.

37th day, Saturday:

There is a lot of worry in the family. I would like to help my mother, but I cannot bring myself to do it, since I would like to break out from under my family's spell. Otherwise, I will not be able to continue to develop myself.

38th day, Sunday:

At exactly 5:00 A.M. I wake up. I had a bad dream that my father died. Does this have anything to do with the worries I have concerning my mother?

Evening: the day itself was successful. I have found an apartment, and despite some uneasiness, I am very optimistic and confident about the future.

39th day, Monday:

No change.

40th day, Tuesday:

I feel light and unencumbered and am hoping for the best, despite outer negative circumstances. Of note is the overpowering feeling that something has been liberated.

41st day, Wednesday, January 11:

For a couple of days now, I have felt a bracing or tightening on the right side of my face. Speaking seems to be a little more difficult.

Besides that, every now and then I feel a tightening under my right breast and armpit.

Despite the many negative aspects, I feel relaxed and, in a peculiar way, I am confident. It seems as if this is an unreal transition phase and I am a spectator to my own situation.

42nd day, Thursday:

Similar to yesterday.

43rd day, Friday:

Actually a black day. Somewhat depressed and off balance. Despite all this, in the background there is rock-hard confidence regarding the change and bettering of my life.

44th day, Saturday:

Similar to yesterday, with a more pronounced positive attitude.

45th day, Sunday:

I have lived very consciously today. I am in a very positive mood and, more than ever, I feel that I am an individual, even someone special.

46th, 47th, and 48th days:

I am restless, am searching and cannot find anything. I want to scatter myself; I am on the run from myself, and cannot come to rest.

49th day, Thursday:

The restlessness subsides somewhat. I realize it is silly to let life pass you by because of fears, for we become successful because of how we deal with experiences. I know everything will happen naturally, cannot be forced.

50th day, Friday:

I have become very calm. I am aware that I need this relaxation phase to gather strength for what is coming up. I sense that something is approaching. Even the outer conditions seem to point to that: the move from my parent's house into the unknown. I know this is only a transitional phase, and I should use it to gain new insights that will help me in the future.

51st and 52nd days:

Despite all that's coming, I do not get into a panic or hysteria—as was the case in the past. I feel at peace and trust God to help me and be by my side, even if I have to cry every now and then. I know that this is a task that I can't run away from or close my eyes to, but which I have to complete. As peculiar as it sounds, somehow I am glad to have a task to accomplish, even if it is hard and not very delightful. Inwardly I am full of confidence and trust.

53rd day, Monday:

Confident.

54th day, Tuesday:

No change.

55th day, Wednesday:

I am not so cheerful anymore. I can't seem to be able to organize myself. I feel separated from other people, so superior, because now I have such a comprehensive view of life, unconfined by time and space. Altogether, though, I feel pretty well.

56th day, Thursday:

I am depressed and listless. I don't feel good. I am all alone. However, I had a beautiful dream: I had my period.

I wish that was really true, because then I would have something that would give me courage to go on. This is the end of the first intake phase.

The prescription for the second intake phase was Walnut and Centaury for seven weeks. Unfortunately, during this phase the patient did not keep a detailed log anymore. The following notes were written down at the end of the seven-week prescription and after the onset of her period.

In this new phase I have not actually discovered anything new about myself. Perhaps I did wish for the reintroduction of my period a little more than before, but I haven't constantly thought about it, just more often than before I started taking the Bach Flowers. A few times I had dreams about this subject. I dreamt that my period came and I had very detailed recollections about my reactions. Sometimes there were sexual experiences in my dreams. More than ever, I have come to grips with my womanhood. A reconditioning of my normal state is no longer out of reach, even if I don't try to attain it feverishly. I am certain that my womanly functions will reinstate themselves as soon as I have found and accepted myself.

Inwardly, I have also disposed of a barrier—the belief I had that my non-menstruating state would never change. This was a thought that I had more or less accepted earlier.

On Saturday, March 10, the third day before the end of the seven-week prescription, I got my first period in six years. It wasn't very strong, but it lasted almost four days. Now I hope that my menstrual cycle will normalize and become more regular. I also hope that the Bach Flowers will continue to help me on my long road to self-determination in the future.

From these notes, one principle of the Bach Flower Therapy becomes apparent: a flower can be introduced only when the time is right. Without the primary treatment phase that dealt with the dissolving of shocks, feelings of guilt, inner fears, and faulty decisions, the final breakthrough would not have been possible. The urge to introduce certain flowers earlier than recommended should be resisted.

Considering the many case studies presented in this book, one should remember the views expressed in Chapter 2. Bach Flower Therapy is a highly individual form of therapy. As there are no two identical people, there are no two identical courses of therapy. The choices and details of the previous case studies should be regarded as examples and suggestions and not as standards by which to make decisions about one's own therapy or the responses of others to therapy.

APPENDIX 1

THE GOAL
of Bach Flower Therapy

The Bach Flowers are thirty-eight subtle, specific, harmonious energy frequencies, obtained by infusing flowers in springwater to form liquid solutions charged with subtle plant energies that act as catalysts and influence the human energy field. The thirty-eight flowers, from wild plants and trees of "the higher order," correspond to thirty-eight specific emotional energy potentials (archetypal concepts of the soul) in the human energy field.

The goal of Bach Flower Therapy is the reharmonizing of the personality's negative moods (fear, mistrust, inferiority complexes) that hinder the emotional and spiritual development of the personality and also trigger physical illness. This brings about a reconnection to the being's God-like core and through it the releasing of a deepening of consciousness, raised self-awareness, and increased self-recognition, self-development, and self-healing.

APPENDIX 2

THERAPEUTIC DEFINITIONS
of Dr. Edward Bach

Soul: The undying part of ourselves, the God-like core of our being, our connection with the cosmos.

Functions as Higher Self, intuition, inner doctor; develops a life plan, lessons, etc.

Personality: The transitory part of ourselves, the character, that presents itself on earth. Realizes the life plan, has various energy potentials (virtues), for example, gentleness, strength to carry through, courage, determination.

Health: The life-plan of the soul realized through one's personality; virtues are being developed.

Illness: Misunderstanding between the intentions of the soul and the insight of the personality, virtues reverse themselves and become deficiencies (cruelty, hate, selfishness, greed). These deficiencies lead to negative moods, fears, bitterness, impatience, and indecisiveness. Negative moods can, in the long run, manifest themselves as physical illnesses. ("It is the spirit that builds itself a body.") This is the soul compensating in an effort to restore the primordially desired state (virtue). The following is an example of the stages of a typical illness and its correction.

STAGE	SYMPTOM
1. Virtue	strength to carry through
2. Deficiency	striving for power
3. Connected negative mood	impatience
4. Possible physical illness as a "correction"	stroke
5. The sick person experiences	unconsciousness
6. He or she has to develop	patience (an aspect of the strength to carry through)

In Bach Flower Therapy, physical illnesses are, at the most, road signs to an underlying malady.

STATES OF THE HUMAN ENERGY FIELD

Health:
"virtues" are being experienced
(positive mood)

- Harmony in the energy field
- The oscillation frequency is correspondingly high
- Filled with psychic energy
- The Higher Self, intuition, or the inner doctor is effective
- Continuing personality development

Illness:
"deficiencies" are being experienced
(negative mood)

- Energetic blockade or distortion
- The oscillation frequency is slowed down
- The psychic energy flow is limited
- The Higher Self, intuition, or inner doctor are hindered
- Inhibited or distorted personality development

Corrections of the Bach Flowers
(virtues reachieved; reconnection
to one's own God-like core)

- Overflowing of the blocked or distorted flower energies by the harmonious flower energy
- Frequencies
- The slowed oscillation frequency is accelerated and reharmonized with the energy field
- The blocked psychic energy is being liberated
- The Higher Self, intuition, or inner doctor can become effective again
- Personality can further develop

Appendix 3

A Step into the Future

Bioenergy Radiation of the Bach Flower Essences

The observation and evaluation of so-called "fine material" healing methods requires, by the natural sciences and others, a visual representation of the energy-information of such methods, in reproducible form if possible. A first, promising step is the color-plate system, developed by the German engineer Dieter Knapp as a refining of Kirlian photography, a system by which the following photographic examples of Bach Flower essences are presented: Star of Bethlehem, Pine, Cherry Plum, Holly, Scleranthus, White Chestnut, Chestnut Bud, and Centaury.

The system involves placing a tiny drop of Bach Flower essence onto a special film. This method has shown that each of the thirty-eight flower essences has a distinctive, characteristic bioenergetic radiation pattern. A renewed photographic record of the same essence taken from a different bottle showed, in principle, the same radiation pattern. For a technical registration of the results, all photographs were scanned with a laser beam. The signal obtained through a photo cell was transmitted via a computer to a recorder that printed the results, presented on pages 91–92. Again in this procedure clearly differentiated and characteristic diagrams resulted for each flower essence. If an objective scientific interpretation of these photographs and diagrams becomes available in the future, it will be added to the collected experiences of Bach Flowers. For today, however, those who are more expert in the flower essences can subjectively make some interesting observations.

For example, it turns out that the radiation pictures of the flowers that mainly affect the mental sphere, such as Scleranthus and White Chestnut, show crisper, more pronounced structures, whereas the photographs of the flowers affecting the emotional planes, such as Pine and Star of Bethlehem, show hazier structures.

Flowers with weaker energetic potential, such as Centaury, Pine, and Star of Bethlehem, manifest themselves in weaker optical forms as well, whereas the more powerful energetic potentials of Cherry Plum, Chestnut Bud, and Holly are represented equally as strong in photographs. Those powerful essences with a slowed dynamic, such as Cherry Plum and Chestnut Bud, reveal such a dynamic in their photographs.

The observation of the color spectrum of these radiation patterns is also interesting. The palette of indigo-blue to pink-red-violet can be found in esoteric representations of healing energies as well.

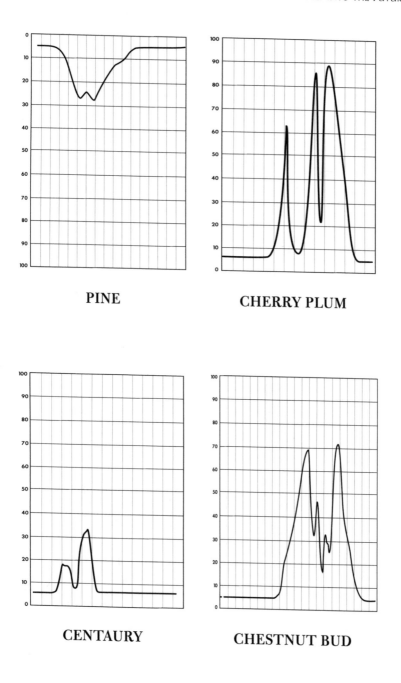

PINE

CHERRY PLUM

CENTAURY

CHESTNUT BUD

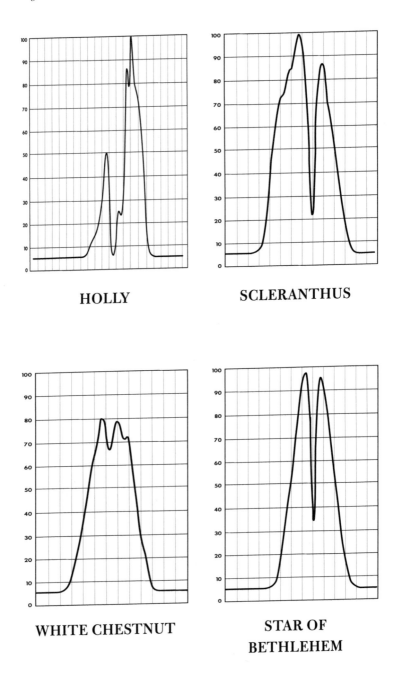

HOLLY

SCLERANTHUS

WHITE CHESTNUT

STAR OF
BETHLEHEM

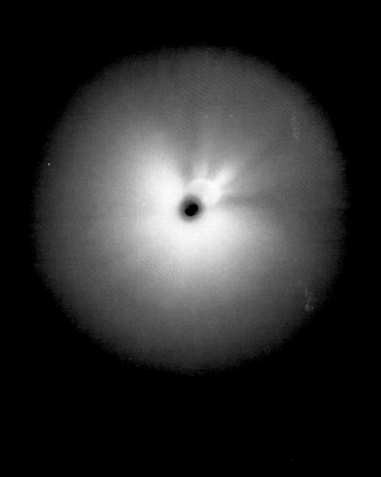

PINE

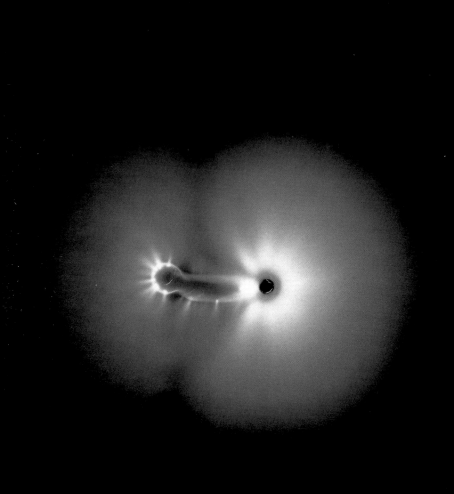

CHERRY PLUM

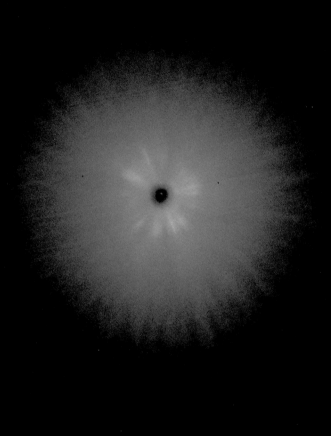

CENTAURY

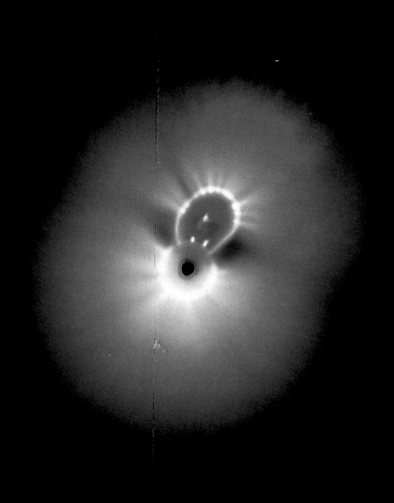

CHESTNUT BUD

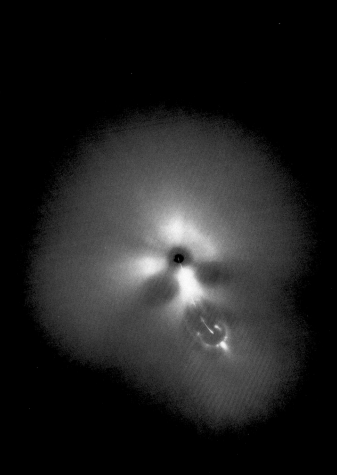

HOLLY

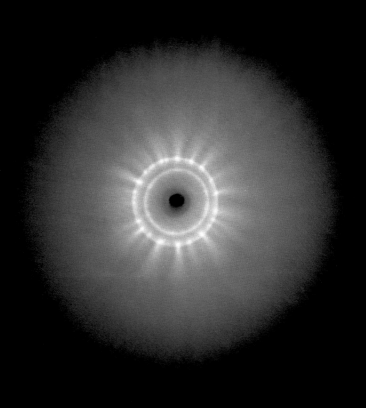

SCLERANTHUS

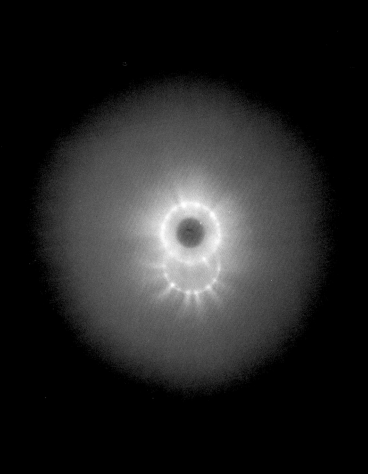

WHITE CHESTNUT

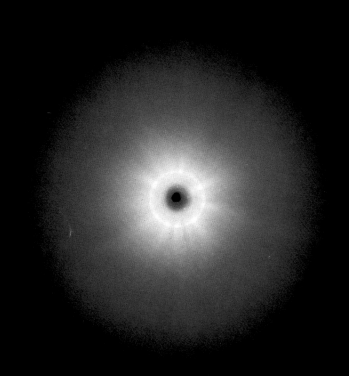

STAR OF BETHLEHEM

APPENDIX 4

DEFICIENCIES CURED
by the Thirty-eight Flower Essences

1. Agrimony—The attempt to hide tormenting thoughts and inner restlessness behind a facade of cheerfulness and a carefree attitude.

2. Aspen—Unexplained, vague fears, premonitions, dread, feelings of an impending disaster.

3. Beech—Intolerance, arrogance, finding fault and condemning others without relating to them.

4. Centaury—Weakness of one's own will, overreaction to other's wishes; your good nature is being exploited; you can't say no.

5. Cerato—Lack of faith in your own opinion.

6. Cherry Plum—Inner fear of letting go; fear of losing your mind; fear of emotional short-circuit; wild temperamental outbursts.

7. Chestnut Bud—You make the same mistakes all the time, because experiences are not properly processed and lessons are not learned from them.

8. Chicory—Posessive personality, always critical and overly inter-fering; expecting your environment to cater to you.
9. Clematis—Daydreamer; thoughts always elsewhere; paying little attention to what goes on around you.
10. Crab Apple—Feeling dirty inside and out, unclean, infected; detail oriented; the cleansing flower.
11. Elm—A passing feeling of not being up to the task of responsibility.
12. Gentian —Skeptical, doubting, pessimistic, easily discouraged.
13. Gorse—No hope, complete despair.
14. Heather—Completely self-involved, always needing an audi-ence, "the needy child."
15. Holly—Jealousy, mistrust, hate, and feelings of envy in all aspects.
16. Honeysuckle—Longing and regrets regarding the past; does not live in the present.
17. Hornbeam—You believe you're too weak to accomplish your daily tasks, but then you succeed nonetheless.
18. Impatiens—Impatient, excitable, overreacting.
19. Larch—Expectation of failure resulting from a lack of confi-dence; inferiority complexes.
20. Mimulus—Specific fears that can be named; dread, "fear of the world."
21. Mustard—Periods of great sadness come and go for no particu-lar reason.
22. Oak—The beaten down and exhausted fighter who continues fighting bravely and never surrenders.
23. Olive—Total exhaustion; extreme physical and emotional fatigue.
24. Pine—Self-blame, feelings of guilt, hopelessness.
25. Red Chestnut—Exaggerated worry and fear for others.
26. Rock Rose—Highly acute feelings of fear, terror, and panic.

27. Rock Water—In the persistent pursuit of particular ideals and principles, other personal needs are repressed.

28. Scleranthus—Indecisive, jumpy; inwardly unbalanced; opinions and moods change from one moment to another.

29. Star of Bethlehem—Aftereffects from physical, emotional, or spiritual shocks, no matter whether they just occurred or lie far in the past; "Comforter of the soul."

30. Sweet Chestnut—Deepest despair. Feeling that one has reached the limit of what is bearable.

31. Vervain—In your excessive zeal to perform a good deed, your powers get exploited; excessively fanatical and irritable.

32. Vine—Domineering, inconsiderate, power-hungry; "the little tyrant."

33. Walnut—Periods of uncertainty, fickleness, and being easily influenced during decisive new phases of life; "The flower that facilitates the breakthrough."

34. Water Violet—Inner reservation, a proud holding back; isolated feelings of superiority.

35. White Chestnut—Certain thoughts run around in your head that you can't get rid of, sometimes including inner discussions and dialogue.

36. Wild Oat—Uncertainty regarding ambitions; dissatisfaction with not having found one's mission in life.

37. Wild Rose—Indifference, apathy, resignation, inner capitulation.

38. Willow—Inner resentment and bitterness; the "victim of fate."

39. Rescue Remedy—First Aid drops. A mixture of Cherry Plum, Clematis, Impatiens, Rock Rose, and Star of Bethlehem. Use after frightful, excitable, or stressful situations.

APPENDIX 5

QUESTIONNAIRE

for the Self-determination of the Correct Bach Flower Combinations

This questionnaire is designed as an aid for doctors, naturopaths, and those who wish to treat themselves, or anyone who has been introduced to the Bach Flower Remedies. It provides a method for understanding the thirty-eight Bach Flower Remedies but should never replace complete diagnostic examinations or a thorough personal self-analysis. Actual use of the Bach Flower Remedies should accompany a basic understanding of the Bach Flower concepts. This questionnaire was developed primarily for the self-exploration of spiritually inclined people in generally good health. (People who are not healthy should fill out the questionnaire with the help of their doctor or naturopath.) The questionnaire should help you recognize which Bach Flower essences might aid in reharmonizing your present psychic state. Each one of the thirty-eight flower essences discovered by Dr. Bach has four questions assigned to it.

Since some states only appear at certain times or in certain spheres of one's life, the questions were separated into 4 groups:

Group 1: Me and My Present Situation

In this case we only refer to conditions that apply to you at the present time, for example the last three days, even if certain traits do not reflect your typical nature (it is possible that in the last three days, in a particular circumstance, you have reacted very impatiently even if this is uncharacteristic. Nevertheless, in this acute state, the essence of Impatiens might be of short-term help).

Group 2 and 3: Me and My Difficulties; Me and My Environment

In these two groups we are dealing with states which, if applicable, will be obvious because they have caused disruption in your life. We are dealing with concepts of negative feelings or emotional misunderstandings that must be dealt with for an increased period of time in order to release the positive energy potential that lays behind them.

Group 4: Me and My Past

This group should help sharpen your awareness of negative feelings you may have believed were under control, but which experience has shown to have been repressed rather than dealt with. These flowers can provide decisive help for future choices of flower combinations as they become relevant in your continuing emotional development therapy.

Please answer every question. Mark the respective questions that apply. Don't skip any questions and don't think very long about your answers. There are no right or wrong answers. It is understandably very difficult to include in such a questionnaire every individually differentiated emotional impulse. Therefore it is possible to come across a question that does not seem to bear any relevance to your situation. In such a case, write the question down and look it over again in a second step, and see if a position can be taken respective to it. If possible, complete the questionnaire by yourself. It should take about thirty minutes, although sometimes takes longer.

Before moving on to the final evaluation of the questionnaire—that is, transferring your answers from the questionnaire to the evaluation table—you should allow yourself a rest period.

Group 1: Me and My Present Situation
(Please answer spontaneously)

	CODE	APPLIES
1. I worry about someone who is close to me.	OR 1	
2. At the time being I feel powerless. I am emotionally and physically exhausted.	QO 1	
3. I am unable to forgive myself for something.	PP 1	
4. I experienced something that has shocked me a lot and I haven't come to grips with it.	KS 1	
5. In the last few days I have been acting more irritable and impatient than is my nature.	VI 1	
6. I have a strong wish to withdraw from something.	FW 1	
7. I am repeatedly bombarded with certain thoughts and images and I can't turn them off.	EW 1	
8. I feel like I'm going mad or flipping out.	HC 1	
9. I have no self-confidence and I tend to be subservient to others.	UL 1	

	CODE	APPLIES
10. I have concrete problems with listening and taking orders.	HV 1	
11. I act carefree and happy to cover up my inner fears and problems as much as possible.	NA 1	
12. I have the feeling that I am very easily influenced and I have to learn to stand up for myself.	KC 1	
13. I am completely discouraged and depressed because things haven't gone as I expected them to.	BG 1	
14. I have to deprive myself of certain things I like.	MR 1	
15. I see many possibilities ahead of me, but I cannot make a decision, which dissatisfies me.	DW 1	
16. I am in a situation that frightens me.	NR 1	
17. I notice that in important situations I get irritated by, and preoccupied with, small matters.	DC 1	
18. In certain situations I feel powerless and at other people's mercy.	BW 1	
19. Other people's stupidity bothers me a great deal.	LB 1	
20. I don't know if my opinions are right anymore.	IC 1	
21. I don't know why, but lately certain things always go wrong.	GC 1	
22. I feel like somebody who's fighting a losing battle, but who continues to fight.	RO 1	
23. I feel melancholic and separated from normal life and feelings, without knowing why.	SM 1	
24. There are signs that I am entering a new phase of my life.	GW 1	

	CODE	APPLIES
25. At this time, I have one or more concrete fears.	TM 1	
26. I don't have the emotional resiliency to handle everyday affairs with confidence.	WH 1	
27. I keep thinking about an experience in my past.	XH 1	
28. I think I am overdoing everything, since I cannot relax anymore.	IV 1	
29. I get my feelings hurt and have difficulty letting go.	YH 1	
30. My situation has no way out; I don't know what to do.	JS 1	
31. Although everything is in order, I feel completely drained, apathetic, with no energy.	CW 1	
32. Because I only want the best for everybody, it hurts me when people misunderstand me.	FC 1	
33. My thoughts vacillate between two possibilities, and I would like to make the decision on my own.	LS 1	
34. I feel overwhelmed by many responsibilities and don't know where to begin anymore.	CE 1	
35. In the last few days I have become fearful. I get into a panic and don't know why.	MA 1	
36. Lately, I have been so busy with my own problems, that I can't recognize other people's problems.	ZH 1	
37. I am pretty discouraged and have barely any hope for a change in my situation.	AG 1	
38. My thoughts are always elsewhere, never here, where they are supposed to be.	EC 1	

Group 2: Me and My Difficulties

(Please do not spend a lot of time thinking about the answers)

		CODE	APPLIES
39.	I always have the same difficulties.	GC 2	
40.	I tell myself everyday: "Calling it quits doesn't count."	RO2	
41.	Although I know what I am capable of, I doubt my capabilities.	CE 2	
42.	When I become disappointed in my positive emotions, they change into the opposite.	YH 2	
43.	I have to admit that I like to get my point across, but most of the time I'm proven right.	HV 2	
44.	Sometimes my own thinking frightens me.	HC 2	
45.	I often feel the need to cleanse myself of something, inwardly or outwardly.	DC 2	
46.	I often feel the need to talk to everybody about myself.	ZH 2	
47.	I tend to feel responsible for other people's mistakes.	PP 2	
48.	I find it difficult to enter a situation or a discussion spontaneously; that is why I would rather stay back.	FW 2	
49.	I have to learn, even more, to be true to myself, even in the face of obstacles.	GW 2	
50.	It makes me antsy when others are very slow. That is why I would rather work alone.	VI 2	
51.	I know that in some situations, I overdo it and virtually roll over others with my dynamics.	IV 2	
52.	I often have a feeling of inner emptiness and of not being a part of anything.	CW 2	
53.	Secretly I have small vices that I don't want anybody else to know about.	NA 2	

	CODE	APPLIES
54. I find truths in many points of view, and always feel compelled to change my convictions.	IC 2	
55. Deep in myself I am unsatisfied because I haven't found my niche in life.	DW 2	
56. I often have panic attacks; I get sweaty hands and have difficulty breathing, a rapid heartbeat, and diarrhea.	NR 2	
57. I would rather achieve most of my goals indirectly.	FC 2	
58. For the time being, I am generally skeptical.	BG 2	
59. Due to exhaustion, I cannot pull myself together, even for things that give me pleasure.	QO 2	
60. I feel I'm a victim of unfair circumstances and I am bitter.	BW 2	
61. I find it hard to say "no."	KC 2	
62. When someone is sick in my family, I always fear for the worst.	OR 2	
63. Unpleasant experiences get played over and over again in my thoughts without coming to a conclusion.	EW 2	
64. Outside my house I am fearful, shy, and overly sensitive.	TM 2	
65. I find it difficult to say to myself: "Don't give up hope."	AG 2	
66. I tend to dwell on the past.	XH 2	
67. More often than most, I reach the limits of my burden-carrying capabilities.	JS 2	
68. I am very strict with myself and am always denying myself something.	MR 2	
69. There are times when I actually enjoy my sadness.	SM 2	

	CODE	APPLIES
70. As early as morning, before I even get out of bed, I have doubts as to whether I can tackle the day; when things get underway, it gets better.	WH 2	
71. I often daydream; as a child, I was not always here.	EC 2	
72. Unpleasant feelings and experiences stay with me for a long time; I have trouble disposing of them.	KS 2	
73. Because I always believe in advance that I will not be able to accomplish something, I don't even attempt it.	UL 2	
74. I notice other people's weaknesses immediately.	LB 2	
75. Very often, for no particular reason, I have an unexplainable feeling of fear and danger.	MA 2	
76. Because I get irritated by outside stimuli very quickly, I always lose my inner balance.	LS 2	

Group 3: Me and My Environment
(Again, please answer spontaneously)

	CODE	APPLIES
77. Others tell me that I get irritated very easily.	RO 3	
78. I am often told that I am too critical and that I should be more tolerant.	LB 3	
79. I have resigned myself to what the future holds for me.	AG 3	
80. I don't think people do anything without considering what they have to gain from it.	FC 3	
81. I often don't trust my own sense of judgement and put more value on other people's opinions.	IC 3	

	CODE	APPLIES
82. Life has withheld a lot from me; I find that unfair.	BW 3	
83. My friends make fun of me because of the stern principles by which I conduct my life.	MR 3	
84. What I admire in others, I don't dare do myself.	UL 3	
85. Feelings of jealousy, revenge, and gloating are best held inside.	YH 3	
86. I sense very quickly when people expect something of me, but I still cannot bring myself to accomplish it.	KC 3	
87. I suddenly become uncomfortable with certain people or in certain surroundings.	MA 3	
88. People around me know that I blow up very quickly, but also that my anger subsides just as fast.	VI 3	
89. Inwardly, I don't wish to commit to anything, which is why I get myself into uncomfortable situations.	DW 3	
90. It is better not to show one's own feelings or vulnerabilities.	NA 3	
91. I have often thought certain tasks were overwhelming but somehow managed to finish them.	WH 3	
92. I am often told that I think only of myself and my own problems.	ZH 3	
93. I often find myself thinking how nice it would be to change something that happened in the past.	XH 3	
94. Everything around me has to have a certain order, which is why I get lost in minor details.	DC 3	
95. I like to keep my distance in dealing with other people.	FW 3	

	CODE	APPLIES
96. I have noticed that I tire much easier than other people around me.	QO3	
97. My friends have told me that in my excitement over a new idea, I can be a little fanatical.	IV 3	
98. Some people are so arrogant that I would rather do the opposite of what they say, even if they are right.	HV 3	
99. From time to time I am overcome by melancholy which passes as quickly as it began.	SM 3	
100. I am told that I make the same mistakes over and over again.	GC 3	
101. At times I have the feeling that my thinking apparatus is overloaded.	EW 3	
102. The brashness of some people hits me very hard and makes me lose my speech.	KS 3	
103. It is possible that I haven't quite broken free of someone who is close to me (mother, father, partner, grandfather . . .).	OR 3	
104. Often there are occasions that make me panic.	NR 3	
105. Life has taught me to give in to what fate has in store.	CW 3	
106. Those around are surprised when I lose control.	HC 3	
107. When I am sick, depressed, or exhausted, I feel like I should apologize to those around me.	PP 3	
108. I lose my balance very quickly; my moods change much more quickly than those of the people around me.	LS 3	
109. I am very familiar with the feeling of having my back to the wall and believing that nobody can help me.	JS 3	
110. I am easily embarrassed when I have to speak in front of strangers.	TM 3	

	CODE	APPLIES
111. When following my own principles, I have to make certain not to let myself be influenced or shaken up by others.	GW 3	
112. Everyday things interest me only marginally. Fantasy has a big part in my life.	EC 3	
113. I tend to overextend myself because I don't want to let other people down.	CE 3	
114. I am being told that I need to be more confident, anchored and to have more faith.	BG 3	

Group 4: Me and My Past

(Please think a little longer about
your answers in this section)

	CODE	APPLIES
115. In school I felt like a failure compared to my fellow classmates.	UL 4	
116. The word "responsibility" played an important part in my upbringing.	CE 4	
117. I had learning problems in my first years of school.	GC 4	
118. As a child, I gladly helped with housework.	DC 4	
119. I had considerable difficulty deciding on a job.	DW 4	
120. I used to have trouble falling asleep, because I had so many thoughts running around in my head.	EW 4	
121. When I look back at my life, I realize that I always got myself into emotional, borderline situations.	JS 4	
122. As a child, I was so emotionally attached to my relatives that I would experience their distress, as if it were my own.	OR 4	

	CODE	APPLIES
123. In my youth I enjoyed taking control, and I always kept a cool head in a crisis.	HV 4	
124. The circumstances of my birth and early childhood were difficult.	CW 4	
125. As a child in school, I always did everything at 150 percent, otherwise I didn't feel good.	IV 4	
126. Even now I dream about shocking experiences that happened years ago.	KS 4	
127. I used to be quick-tempered and furious.	YH 4	
128. Even as a child, I had a weak, nervous constitution.	NR 4	
129. I have built my life on solid principles.	MR 4	
130. My life has always alternated between phases of great productivity and extreme exhaustion.	QO 4	
131. In school I used to enjoy proving others wrong.	LB 4	
132. For a time as a child, I used to walk in my sleep day or night.	EC 4	
133. Fate has dealt me a bad hand.	BW 4	
134. My mood has always oscillated between jubilation and distress.	LS 4	
135. There were people who tended to be depressed in my family.	SM 4	
136. As a child, I was so restless at times that I could not sit on a chair for long.	VI 4	
137. From early on I looked at things in my own way, differently than those around me.	GW 4	
138. In my youth I often had bad impulses that required a lot of self-control.	HC 4	
139. When I was a child, bright lights, shrill colors, and certain noises gave me physical pain.	TM 4	

	CODE	APPLIES
140. I've noticed that without a cup of tea or coffee, or some other stimulant, I cannot begin to work.	WH 4	
141. For the sake of peace I have made a few sacrifices.	NA 4	
142. In my youth I was often confronted by chronically ill people or had a chronic illness myself.	AG 2	
143. During classroom work, I have often crossed out a correct answer and put down an incorrect one—only because of uncertainty.	IC 4	
144. As a child I had nightly fears and strange nightmares.	MA 4	
145. When I was a child I would get an idea in my head and would even use trickery in order to accomplish my goals.	FC 4	
146. Skepticism and pessimism were rampant in my family.	BG 4	
147. I have fewer memories about my childhood than most people.	XH 4	
148. Even as a child I had a tendency to get a guilty conscience.	PP 4	
149. I used to participate in conversations—even if I did not know anything about the subject matter—just to feel involved.	ZH 4	
150. As early as I can remember, I tried to handle things by myself, instead of asking for help.	FW 4	
151. I was a good-natured child. Often I used to do something other than I had intended.	KC 4	
152. In our family it was understood that one would carry a task through to its conclusion.	RO 4	

Final Evaluation

Now transfer the check marks from the questionnaire to the final evaluation table on pages 120–121. With one look, you can see which flower concepts appear most often and which flower essences are being used.

GROUP 1: SHORT-TERM USE FOR AN ACUTE SITUATION

The flowers that you picked out in this group could be helpful to you, on a short-term basis in an acute situation.

It is possible that one or more of these flower concepts normally do not apply to the structure of your character, but in a specific situation are very appropriate.

Favorable mode of application: two drops from each respective stock bottle in a glass of water to be drunk over the course of an entire day. Continue this dosage until the acute state has subsided.

GROUPS 2 AND 3: MIXTURE FOR LONGER USE

Check here to see if in these two groups you have answered one or both statements pertaining to the same flower. If you have chosen the same flower twice, then we are dealing with a flower that, over the next few weeks and months, can be introduced into a regular program for the reharmonizing of emotional states or behavior patterns that have come to a standstill. This flower concept probably relates to the structure of your character. (This also applies if you have chosen a flower in the first group and then once in the second or third group.) The statement is most unequivocal when the same flower is chosen in all four groups.

Also remember that in the beginning it is possible to experience an intensification of negative feelings in the sense of a homeopathic primary reaction. If this happens, try reviewing chapter 2 of this book again.

The flower essences from these groups are best mixed in this manner: two drops from each stock bottle placed in a twenty- to thirty-milliliter bottle, with three parts mineral water and one part cognac, alcohol, or fruit vinegar as a preserver.

From this mixture you can take four drops four times daily, until you decide they are no longer needed. Depending on the situation this could last from four weeks to four months.

GROUP 4: FLOWERS THAT BECOME IMPORTANT LATER.

The flowers marked here could (but do not have to) become very important during the next few months: think about these concepts, and check again later to see if you really need these flowers or not. If you chose the same flower once in Group 2 or 3 and once in Group 4, then you can add that flower to the "longer term" combination.

At the bottom of the table, write down which flower you want to take at the present time. If we are dealing with a lot of flowers, then you should take the ones for the reharmonization of an acute state (Group 1) separately from the flowers for a longer term harmonization of your character structure (Groups 2 and 3).

What do you do when there are more than six flowers in a discussion at the same time? Check to see which of the respective flowers you have chosen in Group 4 ("Me and My Past"), and give this flower priority over the ones that were not marked in this group.

Since all flower essences work together harmoniously, it is safer in the beginning to have one too many flowers in your combination than to risk missing one that could have a decisive effect. Therefore, especially at the beginning of a Bach Flower Therapy, you can combine more than six—even eleven—flowers in a recipe without worry.

In the interest of all the friends of Bach Flower Therapy, we would like to continue to document experiences with it. Therefore, case studies from professional colleagues as well as reports of experiences from lay people, especially examples of dreams, are necessary and welcome. We would like to thank you in advance for all prospective submissions.

Evaluation Table

Please circle the appropriate answers

	GROUP 1 (SHORT TERM)	GROUPS 2&3 (LONG TERM)		GROUP 4 (COULD BECOME IMPORTANT LATER)
AG : Gorse	AG 1	AG 2	AG 3	AG4
BG : Gentian	BG1	BG2	BG3	BG4
BW: Willow	BW1	BW2	BW3	BW4
CE: Elm	CE1	CE2	CE3	CE4
CW: Wild rose	CW1	CW2	CW3	CW4
DC: Crab Apple	DC1	DC2	DC3	DC4
DW: Wild Oat	DW1	DW2	DW3	DW4
EC: Clematis	EC1	EC2	EC3	EC4
EW: White Chestnut	EW1	EW2	EW3	EW4
FC: Chicory	FC1	FC2	FC3	FC4
FW: Water Violet	FW1	FW2	FW3	FW4
GC: Chestnut Bud	GC1	GC2	GC3	GC4
GW: Walnut	GW1	GW2	GW3	GW4
HC: Cherry Plum	HC1	HC2	HC3	HC4
HV: Vine	HV1	HV2	HV3	HV4
IC: Cerato	IC1	IC2	IC3	IC4
IV: Vervain	IV1	IV2	IV3	IV4
JS: Sweet chestnut	JS1	JS2	JS3	JS4
KC: Centaury	KC1	KC2	KC3	KC4
KS: Star of Bethlehem	KS1	KS2	KS3	KS4
LB: Beech	LB1	LB2	LB3	LB4
LS: Scleranthus	LS1	LS2	LS3	LS4
MA: Aspen	MA1	MA2	MA3	MA4
MR: Rock Water	MR1	MR2	MR3	MR4
NA: Agrimony	NA1	NA2	NA3	NA4
NR: Rock Rose	NR1	NR2	NR3	NR4

	GROUP 1 (SHORT TERM)	GROUP 2&3 (LONG TERM)		GROUP 4 (COULD BECOME IMPORTANT LATER)
OR: Red Chestnut	OR1	OR2	OR3	OR4
PP: Pine	PP1	PP2	PP3	PP4
QO: Olive	QO1	QO2	QO3	QO4
RO: Oak	RO1	RO2	RO3	RO4
SM: Mustard	SM1	SM2	SM3	SM4
TM: Mimulus	TM1	TM2	TM3	TM4
UL: Larch	UL1	UL2	UL3	UL4
VI: Impatiens	VI1	VI2	VI3	VI4
WH: Hornbeam	WH1	WH2	WH3	WH4
XH: Honeysuckle	XH1	XH2	XH3	XH4
YH: Holly	YH1	YH2	YH3	YH4
ZH : Heather	ZH 1	ZH 2	ZH3	ZH 4

Intake form: waterglass	Intake form: bottle	You choose intake form
_____	_____	_____
_____	_____	_____
_____	_____	_____
_____	_____	_____
_____	_____	_____
_____	_____	_____

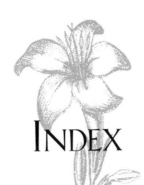

INDEX